# Moral Power

**Series:** Epistemologies of Healing

**General Editors:** David Parkin, Fellow of All Souls College, University of Oxford and Elisabeth Hsu, Institute of Social and Cultural Anthropology, University of Oxford

This series in medical anthropology will publish monographs and collected essays on indigenous (so-called traditional) medical knowledge and practice, alternative and complementary medicine, and ethnobiological studies that relate to health and illness. The emphasis of the series is on the way indigenous epistemologies inform healing, against a background of comparison with other practices, and in recognition of the fluidity between them.

# Moral Power

## The Magic of Witchcraft

Koen Stroeken

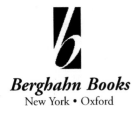

**Berghahn Books**
New York • Oxford

First published in 2010 by

**Berghahn Books**

www.berghahnbooks.com

©2010, 2012 Koen Stroeken

First paperback edition published in 2012

**Library of Congress Cataloging-in-Publication Data**

Stroeken, Koen.
    Moral power : the magic of witchcraft / Koen Stroeken.
      p. cm. -- (Epistemologies of healing)
    Includes bibliographical references and index.
    ISBN 978-1-84545-735-8 (hbk.) -- ISBN 978-0-85745-659-5 (pbk.)
    1. Witchcraft. I. Title.
    BF1566.S7916 2010
    133.4'3--dc22

                                   2010018547

**British Library Cataloguing in Publication Data**
A catalogue record for this book is available from the British Library
Printed in the United States on acid-free paper

ISBN 978-0-85745-659-5 (paperback)
ISBN 978-0-85745-660-1 (ebook)

# Contents

# List of Figures

# Acknowledgements

In a book that has several key players exhorting us to face our indebtedness and learn to live with it, the author should have no difficulty showing deep gratitude, and more. *Wabeja*, Paulo Makufuli. If I may translate the Sukuma formula of thanks: you 'made' me. As did your classificatory father, Lukundula. Maria. Rosi. *Wabeja*. The healers Seele, Doto, Kulwa, Ng'wana Chonja, Ng'wana Mawe and all our neighbours from Wanzamiso. What would this book have been without you? Ng'wana Kapini, now our ancestor, may you rest in peace. Ng'wana Hande: that your dance in tears may continue to carry the spirit.

I am indebted to Mwendesha Sengasenga and his entire family. To Kwiligwa. My teacher Mzee Nzagamba from Nguge: that your novel be printed and widely read. My first teacher, Mzee Pastori Munyeti. My younger brother, Ndaki Munyeti for his unceasing enthusiasm to join us on our mad endeavours. So many others from Misungwi for the friendship in hard times. Let me quickly add, and not be cursed for the many I forgot: Manase Katarayha, Mzee Sakafu, Mzee Doto, Mama Nyanda and her son Peter, Charles, Sjack and Ab, Mama Dogani, Sosthenes, Docta Kinasa, Solile from Iteja, King Kaphipa. What's the point of continuing the list?

Comprehending another epistemology of healing is a never-ending task. For their patience, I thank the Fund for Scientific Research (FWO) in Flanders, the main sponsor of my research. I am grateful to Ghent University for having me continue that work. Presses I should acknowledge include the University of Arizona Press, for chapter 6 reworks my paper 'In Search of the Real' from the book *Divination and Healing* (2004), and also the Journal of the Royal Anthropological Institute, for chapter 8 reinterprets my paper '"Stalking the Stalker"' (2006). Many thanks are due to Mark Stanton and his team at Berghahn for turning my manuscript into a book.

There have been teachers back home. There is nobody like Per Brandström when it comes to thinking through concepts, Sukuma or other. *Wabeja, baba.* Experts on the spirit continue to be Geert Stroeken and Wim van Binsbergen. My deepest gratitude goes to René Devisch, who supervised my research and believed in it from the start. For their valuable comments over the years on parts of this book I should thank, among many others, Bruce Kapferer, Andrew Lattas, Dick Werbner, Peter Geschiere, Knut Rio, Michael Jackson, Michael Lambek, Terry Evens, Olaf Smedal, Philip Peek, Elisabeth Hsu, Annelin Eriksen, Simon Coleman, Sverker Finnström, Karin Barber, Ferdinand De Jong, Einat Bar-Cohen, Paul Bottelberge, Tie Roefs, Don Handelman and Galina Lindquist. Unceasing inspiration and challenging thoughts came from Frank van Lierde, Sophie Stroeken, Wout Quaethoven, Dirk Maetens, 16, and my beloved Annika Waag, to whom I would have dedicated this book had its content been different.

# Preface

In May 2000 I returned to Tanzania for the first time to visit the people I had lived with during two years of fieldwork between May 1995 and June 1997. One of them was my first host and dear friend Butale. (The reason why I choose a fictitious name will soon become clear.) As the shaky drive down to his compound came to an abrupt stop, I found myself surrounded by acres of arid fields, sporadically dotted with stalks of dried maize. It had been an extremely bad year for farmers in this valley. The compound was ominously quiet. With pounding heart I entered but found nobody home. There was no fresh cattle dung and all the houses were deserted, even the large round adobe house where Butale used to live. One rusty shutter, moving in the wind, carried a chalk message written by his son: Do not enter without knocking. The command in the national language of Swahili was very unlike the serenity of Butale and the family I used to know. While I had naively expected to pick up the thread where I had left it, here glowed the embers of disaster, the sort I had studied three years ago, in other places.

In a daze I left the deserted compound and drove up to see Butale's eldest daughter, who was married to a teacher and lived in the school grounds at the outskirts of the village. There we sat in the sweltering heat of her living room, the iron roof creaking under the midday sun. After a long pause, she spoke: 'It happened last year. Father died suddenly. Soon after, his brother died too. The rest of the family had no choice but to move to another village down south'. When I could brace myself to ask her what had exactly happened, she stopped her silent sob: 'I cannot hide this from you. It was witchcraft. In the stomach. They were poisoned'. I pictured Butale before me, a slender, tall elderly man with a gentle low-pitched voice and calm composure. In his openness to my many questions and in his down-to-earth attitude to traditional beliefs, he had come to represent for me the serene balance which many Sukuma farmers managed to attain amidst contradictory pressures from clan, village community, Churches, school and government.

Perhaps the yellow raincoat sealed Butale's fate. That obnoxiously trivial thought about a little gift of mine was the first thing that came to my mind. I had never told the man how much I admired him, how much his unceasing patience and good spirits had pulled me through in times of doubt. For six months I had been his guest, pupil and adopted son, if you will, until the rains came in early 1996, filling the riverbeds around his village and forcing me to find another research location that was accessible by vehicle. When I visited him in the dry season, I gave him a set of waterproof clothes. He visibly approved of the gift: 'Now we won't be cold when herding the cattle during the rainy season'. He had so often told me about the problem before, and what he wanted. The shiny yellow colour of the plastic coat worried me a little though, since it did not exactly blend in with the austere clothing of the other farmers. The image of Butale in his yellow raincoat standing out in the valley now haunted me. Perhaps for his so-called witches, but in any case acutely for me, it was the symbol – as in the Greek *sumbolon*, 'thrown together' – of a larger problem.

A gift that cannot be circulated has the sinister quality of isolating the recipient. Did I ever manage to belong to the gift system in the eyes of his co-villagers? If not, my gift had unduly enriched Butale, which causes jealousy. The jealousy of others that may be a source of pleasure for oneself also raises questions about one's morality, especially in cultures where solidarity is highly valued. One may despise the jealous but one cannot exclude the possibility that their despicable emotion has a moral reason. I am thinking of the Maori notion of the *hau*, legendary since Mauss's study on the gift in 1925, which denotes the spirit of the donor attached to goods. The *hau* haunts the recipients who refuse or fail to reciprocate and who thus have unduly enriched themselves. Debt can mean death. Among the Sukuma patients in the healer's compound where I had worked, the wrath attributed to ancestors was informed by this harsh logic of compensation. In the old days an ancestor weighing on the descendants was considered a curse, called *njimu*. Was the reproach of a witch that different? Both witch and cursing ancestor are thought to feel neglected, jealous of the other's good fortune. Both have moral power in relation to the victim. This, the ethnography will show, is why magic 'works'. The witchcraft in magic is what kills. This foreboding location of disenchanting moralism within enchanting potions of power should unsettle recent scholarship, I argue, for witchcraft and magic are more and more used interchangeably, while the ethnographic depth of initiation that could bring out the experiential nuances between the two is waning dramatically. Anthropology's central themes of gift and witchcraft converge in the moral of misfortune, the jealousy of others, the guilt experienced and reworked. Anyone familiar with healer's compounds will not be led on by occult stories systematically inverting the (hyper-moral) witch into an (immoral) dancer.

The yellow raincoat had little chance of being reciprocated by its recipient. Did the gift to Butale not painfully symbolize my earlier presence, which objectively marked off Butale's compound from the rest of the village? Did it not turn him into *ndoshi*, 'a man full of himself', low in reciprocity and thus bound to be visited by a witch one day? Inadvertently my mind started counting the money in my pocket. I had 80,000 Tanzanian shillings to spare, the value of two cows. But before I could speak, the accusation came. 'You know who is behind it', his daughter said firmly. I was not used to hearing her, the teacher's wife of all people, employ the idiom of witchcraft. Then I remembered that Butale's father, who lived in a neighbouring compound, had remarried. His new wife never gained the family's trust. But this did not make me feel less responsible now. I asked to see her mother. She was staying over at a healer's hospital, in protective custody so to speak, a few villages away. The intense joy of her mother seeing me return after three years left me speechless. Again something totally different was expected than the settling of debts. She did not care about the money. She said she had been waiting for years to see me. Where had I been? I shuddered at the personal feelings taken for granted. 'I am an anthropologist', I wanted to reply.

'What has happened to you?' I could read in their eyes. Did I not remember the times we sweated together in the fields or offering drops of beer and bits of food to the ancestors at the compound altars? What about 'the places' I visited together with healers when opening up the entrails of a bird, entering its beak and descending into the gallbladder to feel our strength and along the stomach to sense out our 'home', mapping worlds I could hardly deny having experienced? Yes, being back in Europe had changed me, three years of extremely volatile, complex and diverse cultural life, all however in one world, remarkably homogeneous in comparison to the places my Sukuma friends and I could move between on just one afternoon in the shade of the tree of the diviner Lukundula.

The one world I was stuck in – call it modernity – strangely suited the bewitchment and the mourning. I felt guilt budding inside me. Clasping some money, I clumsily invented a gift that could translate guilt into something manageable, debt, and end the feeling of intrusion. But here I was, taken aback by the absence of reproach. A monetary transaction could not control our relationship. The clash between transaction and gift was further complicated by a third frame of experience. Butale had once suggested that 'there was a reason' why I, the white man, had wound up in his homestead. While I was preoccupied with my impact, he had considered my intrusion synchronous with his destiny. The intersubjective position I was challenged to take was to not attribute more value to my life story, in which I figured as an intruder among enchanting others, than to Butale's life story, staging himself as the Sukuma receiving an enchanting other. I must admit I found comfort in Butale's reference to destiny. The alternative to feeling bewitched is to accept intrusion (either by oneself or by the surrounding world) as synchronous with one's destiny. In other words, what helped me to escape from the gift system was an experience akin to spirit possession.

This book deals with those two sides of culture: understanding and misunderstanding. On the one hand, cultures have more affinity than ethnographers are often willing to concede. On the other hand, there is something particular about Western modernity in the cultural form it takes, such as schooling and media, whose alterity needs to be pinned down in intercultural terms. From the cultural comparison developed in this book on Sukuma rituals and sensory initiation I learned something about my own culture. I learned that Western modernity is torn between two extreme positions, which I have come to call bewitchment and spirit possession. The split surfaces in the opposition between rationalism and romanticism, and between science and art. Moreover, it surfaces within science itself: between the sciences of nature and those of culture; and within each of these again: between positivist and phenomenological approaches. Modernity's blind spot is the large domain in the middle, where gift and sacrifice interrelate. Here we find the meaning of magic. That blind spot has bedevilled studies of witchcraft, one of anthropology's crown subjects. In those studies we witness the arduous struggle of modern reason asserting the meaning of its imaginary opposite, puzzled by how the concept of the witch is both remote and familiar, almost disturbingly so.

In the first months of my stay when I explained to members of my host institution, a development project, that my purpose was to live in a village and learn about Sukuma culture, they would laugh without exception. The country has an enviable peace record, but subordinating cultural diversity to national unity has for thirty years been part of the *Ujamaa* socialist project. In 1995 when I started my research, culture was something to laugh about. The Swahili word is *utamaduni*, which has the connotation of folklore. Not that the Swahili speaking personnel of the project thought there was no such thing as a socialized set of customs (*desturi*), habits (*mila*) and traditions (*jadi*). But they wished to speak of it as something other people have. (Don't anthropologists as well?). Moreover, this 'culture' the Sukuma farmers had was an obstacle to 'development'; it could never be a resource. Sukuma were associated with a rural lifestyle and witchcraft. How could witchcraft beliefs be a resource? After the laughter came the revealing remark: 'Sukuma are very hospitable but will not let you in on what really matters to them'. The silence on what matters implies two things. In the face of national depreciation of their culture, and of culture in general, Sukuma pay lip service to civil servants and continue traditional practices clandestinely. Secondly, which should interest development specialists and health care professionals, a cultural difference exists within non-Western society that is greater than that with Western society. Therefore, being Tanzanian does not suffice to better comprehend Sukuma culture. Nor does being an anthropologist if current theorizing denies such radical sort of difference for which the concept of culture was originally invented.

In retrospect, my Tanzanian colleagues were right, at least about the first sixteen months of my fieldwork. I realized this after a stroke of luck. The healer Lukundula decided to organize an *ihane* initiation into magic I could participate in. Massively attended by the initiated young men of the valley, it was the first of a series of participations in Sukuma practices I had mistakenly believed to be 'extinct'. For all the unpleasant connotations an ethnographer's initiations have ('going native' for one thing, vanity for another), the conversations afterwards with my fellow villagers radically changed in content and tenor. I had to face the fact that much of the material on magic I had previously collected, as an uninitiated guest, had been mixed with imaginative fabrications sometimes bordering on outright pranks at my expense. I think I can spare the reader the details, and limit myself to saying that some of the witchcraft stories in the media about Sukuma seem instances of that.

This book recounts the six months following my first initiation and subsequent periods of participation when I got more and more acquainted with witchcraft as an idiom of therapy and peacemaking, an idiom somewhat comparable to the way psychology and sociology assist Westerners in coping with contingency. The recent increase of violence and lassitude in the region shall raise the question whether years of institutional attacks on that idiom have not taken their toll on people's capacity to cope with social stresses rising globally. The classification of witches and spirits as religious, or medical, or psychiatric is telling of our own culture. Magic features centrally in Sukuma culture and ties in with so many aspects of social life that its eradication cannot be inconsequential. I will argue that the loss of magical knowledge and practice actually reinforces the figure of the witch and its call for violence.

# Chapter 1
# Introduction: The Meaning of Witchcraft

Sukuma farmers and healers from north-west Tanzania use the word
*bugota* for medicine. The term magic in this book refers to medicine,
yet with an emphasis on the structure underlying Sukuma medicine:
whatever plants are used, at least one ingredient called *shingila*,
literally 'access', should be added to wed the power of plants to the
subject's intention. This ingredient of access, establishing a link which
Westerners would call metaphorical, is required for all potions,
whether for cure, for initiation, for seduction, for business, for
protection or (allegedly) for the witch's sorcery. In magic one can
never be sure of the outcome; that is to say, whether 'access' will be
attained. While *shingila* is what makes magic work, it means accepting
a fundamental instability as a part of life. When asked about the
difference between Sukuma medicine and pharmaceuticals, most
healers point to the *shingila* in their medicine. This complex
combination of a structure, a subjective experience (including an
intention) and access (to a place?) will form the main theoretical tool
in this book.

Whether one calls it a philosophy of life, an epistemology, a
cosmology or, as I do at times, a structure of experience or a state of
the system – and at less verbose moments a place (topos) or a value
– what my fieldwork allows me to differentiate is not Cartesian. It
concerns not what is: mind, body, society, the latter subdivided into
economy, politics, religion and so on, these subsystems themselves
being differentiated into processes I would have discovered. The
distinctions I will offer concern the ways we experience things.
Things come into being because of the human subject experiencing
the world in some way, squeezing the whole as it were through some

1

structure, which eventually delimits a thing (while the specificity of the thing obscures its subjective, holistic structure). Seeing a continuity between the subjective and the social, I will argue that magic stands for one such structure, which permeates rituals of initiation, forms of social exchange and alliance, and not in the least, the open attitude among many Sukuma to their own beliefs in magic. Thus conceived as an experiential structure rather than as a fixed belief, magic questions the definition of modernity as 'living with contingency' proposed by the acclaimed sociologists Beck, Giddens and Lash (1994) in their prominent joint book. Their definition conforms to the self-image of moderns as mankind's tragicomic heroes braving the lure of belief in magical intervention. Does the modern intention, in fact, not divulge the heightened difficulty in living with contingency, with the uncertainty of access to truth? My query does not reproduce the classic opposition of tradition and modernity. It primarily concerns a difference within Sukuma culture. It opposes epistemologically (qua approach to truth) magical practice to the construction of witches.

This introduction tackles the difficulties of such claim about difference. For starters, how could I pretend to capture another culture's practices? That issue lies at the heart of our discipline's 'crisis of representation' (Pels and Nencel 1991), acute since the 1980s and never really resolved. My answer – though I would not claim solution – consists of six brief disclaimers. Firstly, I am after a basic logic or structure rather than 'the' Sukuma culture. Secondly, I am not proposing a Sukuma structure but a structure recognizable to humans at large. My job is anthropo-logy, not Sukuma-logy. Thirdly, since I am not cultureless, the exercise in comprehending culture is necessarily intercultural. The proposed structure will belong to an imagined framework of interrelated possibilities, relevant for my own culture as well. As the example above shows, the concept of contingency can hardly be thought impermeable to Sukuma culture. If not at the level of a concept, contingency is relevant for Sukuma at the level of experiential structure.

Fourthly, there exist several structures in one culture, which can be found in other cultures too (at the abstract level of structures). My starting point is not separate cultures, but what I, as an experiencing subject, recognize in cultures; hence, structures of experience. I am thinking of the moments of affinity I sensed, such as my attunement to the elder protesting against his peers turning spirit mediumship into a business. Very distinct cultural backgrounds and emotional dispositions can converge into places, topoi, which humans move into and occupy together, never exactly at the same spot, but alike position-wise in relation to other possibilities. The cultural diversity authors write about begins with these potentials, which they find within themselves and stimulate. Fieldwork comes in to extend the imagined possibilities and to determine the relative significance of each within the culture experienced. So, anthropologists in practice distinguish at least two dimensions in culture: the people (usually demarcated by a linguistic group) and the possibilities of meaning-making (topoi). Sukuma do not become less Sukuma if the majority of the people actualize other possibilities than they used to.

Fifthly, comprehending culture cannot be done without some form of cultural comparison, translation and structuration of one's own and other people's experiences (cf. Holy 1987; Overing 1987). Therefore, to study structures of experience instead of people's experience itself is, rather than pretentious, a form of modesty as well as honesty about what anthropologists can do with their experiences of culture. We collect and select historical events. I will at times use figures and tables to make explicit the cultural comparisons at work. For much of the differentiation, we may rely on local narratives and reflective exchange with our interlocutors. But some experiential structures are less conducive to narrative reconstruction, while still of relevance to our analysis. For instance, narratives will readily talk of 'modernity' and 'witchcraft' in terms of events such as the conflict or influence between development cooperants and farmers. To realize where epistemological affinities lie takes participation, initiation and other kinds of multisensorial experience. Present studies of witchcraft rely too much on a culture's discourse.

Finally, experiential structures are classificatory rather than natural. In this they are true to Bantu languages and to local approaches to meaning-making, where significant positions in the social network such as fatherhood or sisterhood are always subject to classificatory extension. A Sukuma has many classificatory fathers and sisters. So does an experiential structure include many experiences.

Still, how could the author's experience, however participatory, unravel something as non-subjective as structure? The first thing to realize is that structure is not hard, like a disposition in the body, a module in the mind or a mechanism in society, each supposedly generating (and thus predicting) events. Human structures are soft, for they exist in relations and in the holism of meaning, not in atoms or substances and their impact. As in the aforementioned attunement to the elder's protest despite our divergent backgrounds and emotions, affinity across cultures exists in outcomes, not in origins. A better term for outcome here is meaning. The meaning experienced is what radically disqualifies the mechanistic approach of natural and social sciences. Affinity is in our experience, the thing the fieldworker has close at hand. Therefore it is disappointing in retrospect that globalization studies caused a sigh of relief in the 1990s by in fact keeping our discipline's 'crisis of representation' at bay and replacing the question of meaning and of the author's position by virtually authorless descriptions of historical, macro-social interactions. Ignoring the epistemological relations underlying historical events, I will argue, prevented us from seeing the witchcraft in modernity.

'At the heart of the matter, there is no stuff; only form, only relation', Viveiros de Castro (2004: 484) concludes after listening to pluralist cosmologies both among quantum theorists and among Amazonian Indians. Sheer pluralism is his way of escaping the Cartesian divide haunting anthropology: 'one side reduces reality to representation (culturalism, relativism, textualism), the other side reduces representation to reality (cognitivism, socio-biology, evolutionary psychology)' (ibid.). My interest will be in the reality of representation, notably in the relations that permit representation. I attempt to formulate the relations or structures of representation in terms that concern both Sukuma culture and academic culture. It should be a sign of modesty and reflexivity to limit our unit of analysis in the study of Sukuma culture to the structures by which our interpretation operates. At the same time I admit that this search and reflexivity may increase the introduction's level of abstraction. I hope the rest of the book will make up for these early abstractions prior to interpretation of the data, or inspire a second read. (The impatient reader may want to skip the introduction for now and return to it at the end). The intercultural exercise sets off with my intuition of a complex structure underpinning Sukuma cosmology. It relates gift to sacrifice.

# Gift and Sacrifice (I)

Everything meaningful begins with a severing of the world, the whole, in two, a distinction between something and what it is not. That, at least, is what Spencer-Brown (1969) and Luhmann (1995) posit. I here retain the importance they grant to 'the whole'. Meaning does not come about from combining elementary bits or morphemes, as in Lévi-Strauss's (1962) structuralism, or from adding descriptive layer upon layer, as in Geertz's (1973) interpretivism. Both are textual approaches. Neither fully appreciates the criterion of textual analysis known as the hermeneutic circle, which situates meaning in the relation of part to whole (cf. Ricoeur 1991; Gadamer 2004). Applied to human experience, the non-Cartesian criterion insists on the bodily side of meaning, namely that an experience never emerges in a void but in relation to all the other states the organism has at its disposal. That is the holistic, organic or systemic view of meaning defended in this book. Simplified, one feels sad because one could also have felt happy. Instead, a mechanistic approach concentrates on causality, one module for each experience, as if experiences would not hold together but could be objectively delimited; as if the scientist's meaning itself could do without the system it partakes of; as if the meaning of a thought could be known from teasing apart and reassembling its elementary origins, a mechanistic assumption that Descombes (2001) criticizes about cognitivism. The (Deleuzian) assemblages of DeLanda (2006) attest to the infinite multiplicity of reality, to the micro-level of neurons interrelated with the macro-level of social processes, but they still continue the mechanistic model. What eludes them is how humans perceive the new, as it arrives, giving it a name that structures the whole system at once, which Badiou (2005) names 'the event'. We are looking for such structures that respect the holism of meaning and yet differentiate meanings.

   Where I differ from Spencer-Brown's and Luhmann's holism is in the binarism of semantic distinctions. This is where the contribution of Sukuma cosmology comes in. I should let it come in slowly, as in the Preface, never occluding the cultural comparison at work. It will pay off not to plunge the reader into ethnographic accounts with notions we have fixed ideas about in our own culture such as spirits and witches, too fascinating as entities for us to wonder about the meaning behind them. To avoid repeating mistakes, we have to cast a wider net and tighten it methodically. Then, seemingly similar phenomena such as magic and witchcraft can turn out to have opposite meanings; culturally wide-apart practices such as science and witch construction can appear closely related. Now comes the opening move of our intercultural exercise.

In magic, such as an ingredient whose meaning heals, meaning arises not from a binary distinction, the Western speciality, but from a relation. I contend that the cosmology of Sukuma healers I worked with respects the nonlinearity of events and is therefore underpinned by a relation between two agonistic feelings, the one keeping the other in existence – with an unstability worthy of magical practice and its unsure outcome. What should we call these opposites? Gift and sacrifice are two concepts that seem to percolate through all domains of Sukuma society. While gifts commit the recipient to reciprocity, thus controlling the power balance in society, a sacrifice cannot commit the addressed ancestors. Non-reciprocity may even add to their authority. In magic this difference between gift and sacrifice becomes a relation of interdependence: life is partly sacrificial in that one can never be sure of a return for what one has given (in contrast to the action-reaction of non-magical technologies). Or, just as gifts do not work without some sacrifice of self to the system, sacrifice is meaningless without some expectation in terms of gift logic. Thus, against the many anthropologists for whom 'the gift' since Mauss (1974) answers the perennial question of what keeps societies together, Sukuma cosmology suggests to me that something more needs reckoning: the sacrificial dimension subtending the gift system. The relation between gift and sacrifice expresses the nonlinearity of events, which positivist science fails to evoke.

Within the holistic parameters of my analysis, magic's epistemology will be defined broadly enough to show where it always contains the seeds of the opposite, so-called modern, epistemology. The epistemology has a political dimension. Generally speaking, modern state-organized societies tend to impoverish magical epistemology through specialization. They segregate gift and sacrifice into two worlds, the human and the divine, whereby religion is supposed to establish a grand 'connection', to paraphrase the Latin word *religio*. The mediation of gift and sacrifice is taken out of the hands of the subjects – potential initiands of magic – and out of everyday life. Such reduction of the palette of subjective experience to render members more calculable – for instance on the market – has always interested political organizations governing large communities and territories that escape direct communication and perception. One need not think of Western or modern institutions alone. The conflation of gift and sacrifice is, one could say, the state of the State.

# States of the System: Anthropological Holism

From the above the reader may have gathered my interest in cultural comparison, if not as an aim in itself then at least as a necessary tool for reflexive comprehension of another culture. Cultural relativists would prefer my analysis to stick to Sukuma culture and to particulars about that culture. Their particularism is bound to hit a snag. In surprisingly Cartesian fashion, they are actually expecting me to leave any universalist considerations to scholars of nature, to 'the experts' so to say. Moreover, they forget that there is no way for ethnography to capture 'the' Sukuma. The author offers a cultural version, albeit within an intensified comparative exercise. Finally, every word at our disposal to describe culturally specific events is packed with universality, hence of comparative status. (Even an anti-universalist statement counts on being accessible universally).

When ethnographers manage to 'get into' the culture, they claim to capture a structure of experience, a relation. Louis Dumont (1986: 11, 243–44) warned about cultural traits such as individualism influencing Western expectations about social analysis, as manifested in our tendency to atomize, to grant existence to individuals and elements but not to relations. I will propose that our social theory take its cue from the epistemology of magic. Moderns have learned to disparage four possibilities: of intercultural understanding, of one experiential relation underlying disparate beliefs, of the bodily relevance of meaning, and of the universal accessibility of ritual meaning. Magic is holistic in operating on exactly those four possibilities.

The holism I propose is two-pronged. I show witchcraft to exhibit a logic or structure within Sukuma society that is interrelated with other meaning structures in that society.[1] However, I argue that this structure cannot be separated from a broader system of conditions of possibility pertaining to the human body and society as such. This second step relates the holism of 'a culture' – Sukuma structures of experience – to the holism of *anthropos* – human structures of experience.

Anthropology as the study of humanity is holistic by complementing social, political, economic and biological aspects that other disciplines do not (Parkin 2007: 6). Anthropologists thus acknowledge that cultures are systemic, all parts closely linked within and across cultures, and that cultures are dynamic, continuously prone to social, economic and biological processes, so that a people could not be stereotyped through one transmitted belief or practice, such as witchcraft and witch killing. This book can be read as an ethnographic defence of that culture concept, via the notion of experiential structures as systemic states. Anthropological holism does not, like Richard Rorty's (1989) postmodern hermeneutics, situate holism in meanings forming a whole segregated from the real, from nature 'out there'. Such a hermetic take on meaning is surely too culturalist, too Cartesian for our taste. Nor is it the holism of Marx, granting causality only to social aggregates, with the parts being epiphenomena. Like meaning (versus matter), the social (versus subjectivity) then becomes another Cartesian partition, again shielding off a reflexive question, namely how the author can know those social aggregates.

Integral to our holism's second, intercultural step is that the author's reflexivity, rather than hard data, improve our knowledge when it comes to meaning. The relations of part to whole, making up the meaning of what we study, significantly deepen as we include the author's own relating to the whole. For instance, we learn more about the Sukuma belief in spirits if we take into account the ethnographer's urge to downplay the universal value of this belief and stress its culture-specific aspects in order to keep at bay the cognitivist who might come up with evolutionary mechanisms to explain the surprising fact of a widely occurring belief without apparent empirical grounds (here the existence of spirits). An equally revealing part of the Western author's experiential structure may be misgivings about the spirit element (and other forms of 'superstition') for mitigating the individual's autonomy and responsibility in the world (while Sukuma might appreciate the awareness of such mitigation as more sensible and more socially sustainable, keeping people more cautious and peaceful). These intercultural tensions determine the meaning the ethnographer writes about. None of these aspects of the meaning are mechanisms; they constitute a range of possibilities for viewing the world, which relate to each other and across what could be called 'the system'.

Anthropology uniquely has the grit to study the human, an amalgam of social, economic, political, psychological, biological, medical and other divisions begun by Cartesian dualism and delineating scientific disciplines. Anthropological holism requires we perceive the world at right angles to the way in which other disciplines do. This far exceeds interdisciplinary exchange, for such exchange perpetuates the divisions. Rather, it entails we look at what crosscuts the parallel subsystems under study. I propose we do this by studying the various states the (whole) system can be in. From a Kantian perspective this may look like shifting our focus from theoretical to practical reason; that is, from causality to intentionality (Dilthey's famous pair), or from reality to morality. Assessing the state of the system is indeed a moral act, if we define one state as ill or abnormal and another as healthy or normal. But many cultures do not go for the dualist assessment, otherwise so popular in monotheistic religions (Parkin 1985: xi). The witch's 'evil' is not a simple inversion of social order. The Sukuma witchcraft idiom I picked up in the healer's compound distinguishes at least four interrelated, possible states of the system, which I tentatively describe as reciprocal, intrusive, expulsive and synchronous. The states will correspond to the experiential structures of, respectively, the use of magic, the feeling of bewitchment, the redress of divination and ritual healing, and the experience of union with the intruder through spirit possession. Those bewitched, often to the point of losing their wits, are not socially stigmatized. Instead of being ill versus being healthy, they experience one of the states (more or less intensely) any human can be in. 'The world' they live in has transformed in a certain way, they say. This makes for an attractive methodological stance. The quaternary dynamic of the witchcraft idiom (reciprocal, intrusive, expulsive, synchronous) takes the edge off the moralism characteristic of dualism (good/bad) without however lapsing into the Kantian pretense of value-free assessments about the world.

Famous assessments of states of the system, such as Marx's historical materialism and Habermas's critical theory diagnosing modern capitalism (see Chapter 4), have a certain Western ideal state in mind. Anthropologists working in the postcolony since the 1970s tried to develop the next step after Marxism through what Marcus and Fisher (1986) called a 'cultural critique'. Juxtaposing different cultures would result in a more culture-sensitive analysis of society at large. Exemplary here is Taussig's (1980) portrait of capitalism with its 'unnatural' sociality as seen from the perspective of Columbian peasants' epistemologies. Their Faustian magical response to the plantation economy would be telling in itself as a social critique. I cannot deny that my ethnography continues the search for a non-Western social assessment with greater moral complexity, reassessing our view of society and revealing the premises underlying the mistakes of our ancestors (which we are in danger of repeating). However, my method will not be to start from Western theories such as Marxism, nor to juxtapose two cultures, which would require we objectively represent and neatly disentangle each culture in our experience. Rather, on the understanding that no author is cultureless, fieldwork creates an intercultural platform where the author's culture's terms can meet the other culture's terms (cf. van Binsbergen 2003). That is the mediatory 'third' culture of anthropological analysis (Strathern and Lambek 1998). It combines the modesty and reflexivity I defended earlier. It should inspire caution about analyses that pretend to unravel a particular culture's mentality or 'structure of feeling' (Williams 1975) or, more recently, its 'culture structure' (Alexander 2003). By lack of reflexivity about the author's proper interpretive structure, these notions become objectivist. They magnify the sociologist's paradigm of socialization to the point of cultural essentialization. Anthropologically, a culture may rather refer to a social reality that stimulates certain states (manifest in experiences as much as in social processes) within a range of interrelated possibilities available to all humans. A fascinating example, therefore, in the eyes of anthropologists has always been what healers and diviners do; their reflexivity of commenting on society, thus hoping to improve the state it is in, while initiating outsiders – sometimes from different cultures – into the experiential structures permitting these comments on society's state.

10

# Gift and Sacrifice (II)

Arguably the most significant concept for comprehending culture worldwide is 'the gift', the concept Mauss used to compare societies and which never left the scene unlike anthropology's other fads. Defined not as a universal practice but as a form of social exchange related to other forms such as sacrifice, the gift concerns one condition of possibility for 'society', for people living together, and may therefore be expected to inform people's assessment of states of the system. As suggested in the Preface, witchcraft refers to one such state. Thus we should not be astounded that relations between gift and sacrifice together constitute a semantic framework revealing the meaning of something as seemingly unrelated as witchcraft.

Once scholars from various fields and geographic regions sit together to decide on the meaning of a practice, they often conclude that the definition can be ever extended to the point where it becomes a virtually empty category. The message is that we will always be lagging behind culture's creativity. For example, Signe Howell (1996: 2–4) remarks that the concept of sacrifice is 'too much of a ragbag of elements', and is hence not useful for cultural comparison. The minimal definition of sacrifice she begins with, 'the ritual taking of a life', first lost the element of 'ritual' (because hunting also turned out to be a form of sacrifice), and then 'life' as well (because in one instance money was sacrificed). Such deconstructive outcomes have marked many definitional debates. Howell cites among others those regarding religion, kinship and ritual. The compromise reached in these definitional debates has become almost commonplace: to accept Wittgenstein's 'family resemblances', or Needham's (1975; cf. Shipton 1989) polythetic classification, whereby a variable cluster of elements determines the class to be defined.

Although I agree that no single series of elements can define a concept, it is still atomistic to reduce a meaning to the association of many elementary meanings, as suggested by family resemblances and the polythetic. Sacrifice has elements of religion, giving and violence, but none of these has a fixed meaning either. In anthropological holism we proceed the other way around. We start with the whole – human experience – and progressively differentiate it. So, to define the meaning of sacrifice, we go at least one level up (not down) in classification to compare sacrifice with other forms of exchange. I find three more forms distinguished throughout the literature: commodity, present and the gift, our starting point. I propose the four are 'mutual' opposites that cover the whole of human experience, if in very general terms and limited to the social domain.

The first distinction, between gift and commodity, inspired early social critiques of commodification from the end of the nineteenth century until the mid twentieth century, whereby gift exchange was contrasted with the alienation of social relations in capitalist production. Bourdieu (1980) and Appadurai (1986) later brought a more nuanced understanding to the opposition by noting that gift exchange and commodity exchange both serve people's self-interest. Both forms of exchange operate on the social law guaranteeing the giver's investment. The inalienable character of gifts should not mask their instrumentality in status-production. I shall argue, though, that it is (post)modern to blur the distinction between gifts and commodities. In all cultures, gifts add to the social law of debt and credit the dimension of relationship, which is a combination of at least two aspects: the attention paid ('the thought counts') and a certain duration before returning the gift. The dimension of relationship, constituted by these two aspects, comes down to an acceptance of contingency and lack of control. That is what distinguishes the unpredictable battle of magic and counter-magic from the moral power and law of the witch.

The second distinction partaking of the gift's meaning is the one Mauss made between gifts and 'free gifts', or what I call 'presents'. Presents deny the social law in the gift and idealize the other dimension in gifts: the relationship. The same (e.g., Western) societies that commodify economic exchange appear to idealize the free gift. As Parry (1986) argued, the ideology of the pure gift in world religions (in his case Hinduism) emerges in parallel to the ideology of the individual pursuit of utility. Societies that employ gifts for utility, are considered impure by these religions. The purification, whereby economy and affection are separated, surfaces in Western theories of society – for example, in Habermas's (1985) colonization thesis where he pleads for keeping the two apart (see Chapter 4). Purification is not, like Latour (1993) defines it, a Cartesian separation of nature and society. Purifying gift from relationship, which is what commodity exchange comes down to, is a moral act. It attempts to force morality out of the picture and store it in a safe place, an ideal also found in Kant's opposition of theoretical and practical reason.

The third form of exchange to distinguish from (and relate to) gifts is, finally indeed, sacrifice. Much of the literature on sacrifice can be read as oscillating between two definitions, which Milbank (1995: 89) finds united in Hubert and Mauss's (1899) classic work: sacrifice as a gift to the gods according to *do ut des* ('I give for you to give') and sacrifice as (an often violent) expiation resulting in rebirth. I remark that both definitions understand the violence of sacrifice as an investment. They do not escape the logic of the gift. Thus they fail to comprehend sacrifice other than as a variant on the gift. De Heusch (1985: 7) has likewise criticized Hubert and Mauss, noting that in many societies sacrifice is merely worship, which does not transform the giver's ontological status. I will argue that the person sacrificing does undergo an experiential shift (which is one reason for sacrifice fulfilling an important role in Sukuma therapies), but I agree with de Heusch on sacrifice differing from the gift. I agree to the extent that sacrifice, unlike the gift, does not change the social status of giver and receiver (the gods, ancestors). In other words, sacrifice is a special form of exchange quite complementary to the gift. While sacrifice implicitly feeds the expectation of return (for example, health and prosperity) from the receiver (such as the ancestor), its outspoken meaning is the exact opposite: placation, beseeching the blessing from the ancestral spirits. Spirits are not committed by sacrifice, as receivers in the diurnal world are by gifts. Furthermore, contrary to the accumulation of capital and status through gifts, sacrifice violently destroys what one holds dear. This destruction is a discontinuous practice escaping the calculus of debt and credit, as one would expect from an experience opposite to that of the gift. The Sukuma word for sacrifice is *shitambo*, which is also a term for 'hunt'. I see no better way of referring to an event one can never be sure of.

Gift and sacrifice are opposites yet of the same origin, much like committing the other and submitting to the other are interdependent, constituting the social. Sacrifice is not a mere derivation from the gift. It only becomes that in an anthropology like Girard's (1993) which views humans as driven by self-interest (which he calls desire) and nothing complementing it. Everybody's wish to emulate and possess what others have would result in mimetic

13

violence. Sacrifice of a human scapegoat, typically the witch, would be the cathartic response. The analysis changes radically, I contend, once we grant self-interest a full-blown counterpart. I am thinking of a four-letter word that art, unlike science, abounds with: 'love', the sense of an umbilical tie between self and others, whereby anything affecting the latter will affect the former. Could love be the twin of desire, like sacrifice is of the gift? Our individualist society prefers the romantic picture of love coinciding with desire, or opposed to it, not mixed. Ethnographers working in Sukuma villages have the unfortunate job of explaining to their compatriots what love is like when it is less individualized, less focused on one individual, as in romance, and more diffuse, socially oriented, as much a physical as mental kind of well-being depending more on the group, on the totality of men and women one lives with, and therefore more prone to cause complex emotions such as jealousy within that group. In brief, focusing on desire alone will not help us comprehend witchcraft in Sukuma villages. We have to get love back in the picture. That is what I intend by relating gift and sacrifice.

# Moral Power (I)

The distinction and relation between magic, witchcraft discourse, divination, exorcism and spirit possession have remained remarkably unstudied, perhaps because of the way our secularized minds have lumped these practices together under the rubric of 'religion'. This book elicits their fundamentally social, rather than religious, meanings by studying the forms of exchange they correspond to. Gift and sacrifice stand for distinct ways of relating in ritual (alliance versus worship), in politics (power versus authority) and economy (debt versus duty), among others. The connection between witchcraft and the gift is certainly not new, but its sacrificial counterpart, this invisible dependence felt in relation to the family, the clan and more abstractly the group, has largely been missing in the social analysis of power, witchcraft and social exchange. The anthropological study of sorcery focused on social competition and unlimited desires of powerful politicians or sorcerers boasting about their magic. However, in the healer's compound, in situations where the lifeline is under threat, people's umbilical tie with the group appears. Patients do not feel 'less' power; that is, defeated by a stronger opponent. They feel power-less. The magic that lethally poisons has in itself little explanatory value for those personally facing their death. Patients in the healer's compound ask the existential question: How could my life end, how could my ancestral guide desert me? The battle of magic and counter-magic is not adequate as a perspective for understanding patients inflicted by magic. *Ndagu* – the curse in magic – is what patients and healers alike are concerned with. It is what overruled the ancestral guide's protection and authority and eventually rendered the witch's black magic lethal. The use of magic is an everyday (if discrete) affair. The witch is of another order. To be able to go as far as lift the ancestor's protection, the witch must be entitled to the victim's life. Witches must have a reason, in the two meanings of the word. They must have a motive, such as feeling neglected, and since such a motive would be sufficient for them to go out and kill, they must have a rationality of their own. The witch combines aspects of both morality and power into something foreboding that the witch alone has: moral power. The witch's credit, literally 'eating thing' (*shili*), is what's eating the bewitched.

The most common *ndagu* curse is *ibona*, 'the look'. It refers to revenge: 'You'll see!' as my interlocutors added after imitating the witch's silent stare at negligent kin. We may think of the 'evil eye', or the English expression 'if looks could kill'. What the witch has is neither morality nor power, but both at once. Moral power is not the power of magic, earned by individuals skilled enough to defeat their opponents. Nor is it the authority invested in elders and ancestors, also known as socially recognized power, which permits them to sanction people (to use Weber's classic distinction). Moral power arises at moments of crisis, and lives in suspicions, before these become public accusations. It travels and circulates until it is identified and ritually dispelled.

Pivotal for healers ritually dealing with moral power is the monitoring of their patients' construction of the witch, through divination among others. This construct is not exactly the product of a culture, as in an interiorized, pre-given belief. The idea of the witch arises from a situation, one surprisingly similar to Descartes's primal scene after utter doubt. In the healer's compound among the bewitched we witness the birth of culture, albeit of the least expected kind: the birth of a clear and distinct idea. It is the idea of the witch's identity: 'X is eating me'. The reason attributed to witches for their action is an intense belief emerging from the event of crisis, rather than the reproduction of a traditional belief. The idea is modern in the sense of trusting not in tradition but in the 'recent', *modo*, as the word stem suggests, in what comes up in the here and now of experience. But it is also modern in its content, in the kind of person suspected in terms of kinship, gender and social status. The concrete construct of the witch, probably long predating the arrival of Europeans, shows remarkable affinity with the position of gender specialists today, as it defies traditional norms and duties by conceding that women have been badly treated by the clan system and therefore have sufficient moral power to take the life of the patient, man or woman. I thus speak of 'the ever modern'. Fears of the witch deviate from magic cosmology in that they pervert an idea central to magic: people's umbilical tie with the group, the ancestors and the clan. Our ethnography will illustrate the many ways in which healers' practices incorporate this experience of the ever modern. We are on a collision course with the dominant literature, as the next part of the introduction sketches. Latour's (1993) famous formula will be inverted: we have always been modern – sometimes.

# 'Modernities' and (Dis)enchantment

South of Lake Victoria, in the semi-arid valleys between the Serengeti plains to the east and the hills of Rwanda and Burundi to the west, live agro-pastoral farmers cultivating maize and cassava, rice in good years and cotton as a cash crop. With a population of about 5 million, Sukuma form Tanzania's largest cultural group. Like their Nyamwezi neighbours in the south, who speak a very similar Bantu language, their kinship and inheritance system is structured around patrilineal descent and virilocal (though now mostly neolocal) marriage; the latter ideally involves bridewealth, if not in cattle then in cash. Before Tanzania's independence in 1961, the chiefs or 'kings' (*batemi*) of the fifty or so chiefdoms that to outsiders made up 'Sukumaland' had to collaborate with the British colonial administration in a system of indirect rule, which in this resource-poor part of Tanzania meant quite limited intervention. In the mid 1990s, when I conducted most of my fieldwork, the impact of schooling and Christianity remained relatively minimal. According to Wijsen (1993), the 10 percent

Catholics formed the largest Christian denomination while some 2 per cent of the total population followed Islam. The suggested 80 per cent without denomination reflected the Catholic parishes' strict conditions of membership such as church attendance and abstention from polygamy. This figure does not reflect the widespread knowledge of and sympathy for Christian beliefs. Nevertheless, Sukuma have long been known in Tanzania for being the least interested in proselytizing religions, this despite missionary presence since the 1880s. Varkevisser (1973) claims that in the 1960s about 35 per cent of the population of Bukumbi chiefdom close to the town of Mwanza were Catholics. Christianity has been more successful in the rest of Tanzania, especially in the hilly areas of Arusha, Moshi and Bukoba, which have long attracted white settlers for coffee plantations.[2] These areas also have a milder climate – for example, being less mosquito-infested – making them tourist hubs for visiting the country's national parks. However, the Sukuma plains, south of Lake Victoria, have been left aside by the tourist business.

Most villages have no electricity, running water or public transport, but form open communities, welcoming outsiders as well as foreign goods, especially those that raise connectivity, such as bicycles and radios, and recently mobile phones. Population density and pressure on land are high, so much that adolescents are increasingly pushed out of agriculture and pulled into urban migration. Extended residential families, which are decreasing, live at a distance from each other in rather self-reliant compounds, usually with a cattle pen, surrounded by their fields. Since most of the political, economic and ritual activities occur in or around the compound rather than in the centre of the village, one could speak of a 'polycentric' society.

The idea of ancestors acting as protective spirits is widespread. In the villages of Wanzamiso and Nguge where I worked even the few farmers that went to church would build ancestral altars in their compound to ritually placate the ancestral spirits in the case of grave illness within the family. Village councils rule by consensus, which again leaves the main decisions to the family, usually represented by the oldest man, a grandfather. As will be detailed later, there is probably a cultural reason for the failure of the monocentric model, which Tanzania's socialist administration attempted to implement in the 1970s. Where I lived, the created village centres had a primary school, an office of the ruling party CCM inhabited by the government representative (Village Executive Officer), a cotton storehouse, but not a market and dispensary like in the bigger villages along the main roads. The village centre remained squarely outside village life.

The polycentric village extends into a less visible reality, a loosely structured social network. Since colonial times, and probably before, Sukuma farmers have reproduced an informal politico-medical system consisting of initiatory societies waxing and waning in popularity, healing traditions, innovative magic and spirits, which span central East Africa, from the Great Lakes to the Swahili coast. A beautiful monograph could be written on the history of these initiatory societies, their founders and related traditions in East Africa (cf. Ranger 1975; Gunderson 2001). Here, however, I will concentrate on research that in my view is of still more pressing need: the epistemology of healing constituted by these traditions and societies. It concerns a partly sensorial knowledge which is imperceptibly but increasingly being offset by the premises and values of national and international policies, by media and socio-economic development projects, as well as by the informal intercultural communication we all engage in. Regarding the latter, a pivotal role is played by development and globalization studies that disconnect practices and beliefs from their anthropological (by which I mean both culture-specific and universally relevant) structure, and lament their 'disappearance' or revel in their 'revival', and equate culture with identity.

This study originated in ethnographic fieldwork in Sukuma villages between 1995 and 1997, with return visits in 2000, 2003, 2007 and 2010. As my contacts with healers and their patients grew deeper, so rose my discomfort with existing theories of witchcraft. From studying the creative process of belief construction in healer compounds, I learned that the idea of 'the witch' is central but nevertheless interchangeable with other ideas such as ancestral wrath, the group's sanction and collective gossip, and that the idea the bewitched patient forms of the witch concretizes in certain figures such as a marginal elderly woman isolated from the group and suspected of holding a grudge, figures that have a radically different tenor than that of the magic I readily associated with them. While magic was of an everyday, diurnal kind, and witches were supposed to be nocturnal, one's personal concretized witch was neither: 'the' witch was so utterly diurnal – in the blandest way – and so utterly nocturnal – in the most disturbing way – that one could only wish this person dead. It will take a book to refine the nuances of this difference between magic and the witch. It relies on the experiential dimension of meaning following the phenomenological and interpretive turns of the 1970s, which confronted 1950s-style functionalism for explaining witchcraft beliefs from the perspective of social control. Since the 1990s a new 'ism' has been on the rise that did not heed the critique. Englund (2002) has referred to it as the rhetoric of globalism, an explanation of witchcraft in terms of global forces. The literature ignores a culture's proper distinctions, in service of what is, in itself, an attractive observation, made by Jean and John Comaroff (1993) and Peter Geschiere (1997); namely, that far from being the opposite of modernity, witchcraft seems 'a fixed corollary of modernity' (Fisiy and Geschiere 2001: 243). The observation that witchcraft beliefs are not vanishing under the influence of modernity could have been interpreted as a revealing one for our modern epistemology. It could have paved the way for a debate on the ways in which humans make meaning and assess the social situation they are in. It could have led us to unpack both 'modernity' and 'witchcraft' to the point where one concerned the other. However, something else happened. Globalist studies chose to attribute the ongoing relevance of witchcraft beliefs to the detrimental effect of modernity and the contemporary manifestation of the capitalist economy. As a result, witchcraft lost nothing of the alterity moderns had always attributed to it. A set of traditional beliefs and practices that date from before colonization were treated as a symptom of postcolonial disorder. Might this not be the last thing that we as anthropologists intended?

Have theories of social processes been a way to avoid epistemological discussions, which have seemed unresolved since the crisis of representation? The value of magic as a cosmology is conspicuously absent in the witchcraft literature since the 1990s. In a trenchant critique somewhat tucked away in his comprehensive introduction to witchcraft and magic, Kapferer (2003: 18) argues that in their eagerness to diagnose the postcolonial predicament, authors such as the Comaroffs have been indirectly pathologizing magic, which brings us back to its association with irrationality, something our discipline seemed to have long left behind. The ethnographer's first question should be how witchcraft is integrated into a system of ritual traditions, practices of healing and diagnosis, marriage rules, decision-making and eventually the State and wider social systems. This relational totality, which I call an experiential structure, can hardly have changed overnight with colonization. It has done the study of witchcraft no good to limit itself since the 1990s to the public arena of discourse and politics, far away from the obscurity of the healer's compound and the victim's home where the witch actually comes into being.

A consensus has come to exist since the 1990s that the reason for 'the modernity of witchcraft' is not the resilience of witchcraft beliefs or the flexibility of magical thought, as in the 'secondary elaborations' described by post-evolutionist anthropologists such as Mauss, Evans-Pritchard (1976) and later Horton (1967). Modernity itself is seen as the instigator of witchcraft, because modernity has political and economic implications creating new inequalities between Africans. Jean and John Comaroff (2000) have argued that discourse on the occult in South Africa follows on from the neoliberal course the postcolonial economy has taken. Francis Nyamnjoh (2001) illustrates this in Cameroon where suspicions of sorcery arise from the occult ways in which the market mechanism rewards some and undermines the (traditionally protected) status of others.

The list of similar analyses is extensive. Rumours have it in Tanzania that their Zambian neighbours in the south fare better thanks to magic made from the skins of Tanzanian peasants and sold across the border. Todd Sanders (2001) regards these stories of occult trade as an indirect form of protest against an unsustainable economic situation. The idea can be traced back to Taussig's (1980) study of Columbian plantation workers: their belief that capitalist benefits can only come from black magic and a Faustian contract with the devil reflects their exploitation. The postcolonial elite, especially in Africa, went further in embracing the occult in return for capitalism's benefits. Politics in modern Africa has often come down either to abrupt interventions of an anonymous State in village affairs, or to arbitrary, predatory actions of postcolonial rulers, as unforgettably evoked in the work of Achilles Mbembe (2001). In the wake of decolonization, Mary Douglas (1970) and her contemporaries discussed the possibility that the witch internalized colonial authority, thus suppressing the revolt needed. Twenty years later African rulers themselves appear to incarnate the witch, defined as a figure of insatiable desire and anti-social accumulation – a figure of excess that itself renders the ruler immune to critique and thus more powerful (Bayart 1993). A large part of the African continent suffers from structural violence and inequality, which would result in witchcraft beliefs gone awry, the prime example being witch hunts (e.g., Ashforth 2001; Niehaus 2001a). In brief, Evans-Pritchard (1976) once argued that speculations of witchcraft serve to explain misfortune. Today a host of researchers have extended the concept of misfortune to social inequality.

This is how magic can appear as a 'corollary of modernity'. The other direction of argumentation has been explored as well: modernity as magical. The study of witchcraft would have risked being deserted by now out of embarrassment over the scholarly fascination with such non-modern epistemology, or shunted to the bookstore's New Age section, had the authors cited above not revived it since the 1990s with a double, counterintuitive twist challenging the epistemological dichotomy and hierarchy between modernity and tradition. Not only is witchcraft a logical response to modernity, modernity itself is all about enchantment. The claim is that society has not been increasingly rationalized or 'disenchanted' as Max Weber (2002) predicted a century ago. Modernity's economy, media, science, technology and politics draw on the enchantment of large audiences. Modern artefacts and knowledge enchant newcomers, often after these objects appear as enchanted themselves. Moreover, religion, enchantment in the strict sense, abounds across the globe more than ever and in many forms, old and new. Are witchcraft beliefs not one of these religious forms responsive to modernity's enchantment? A new consensus has emerged across the social sciences and humanities that we should stop speaking of modernity in the singular, given its implicit opposition to tradition, and to magic. Rather, we should acknowledge the plurality of 'modernities' populating the planet today (Moore and Sanders 2001; cf. Gaonkar 1999; Taylor 2004). As Englund (1996) argues, the Comaroffs were probably the first to broaden the concept of modernity so as to have it contain all kinds of magic, rather than oppose modernity to magic and propose a process of transition from the latter to the former (as Taussig did, Englund argues). They granted each non-Western culture its non-Western modernity. But, Englund argues, they should have taken the next step and have each modernity fill in its own magicality, including normative decisions on what is occult: Englund gives the example of individualist versus reciprocal accumulation of capital in Malawi, where merely the former is deemed occult.

What all those authors share, I argue, is a broadening of our concept of modernity and of magic in a theory of plural modernities and magicalities, which duly breaks with the dichotomy of modern/ traditional, yet unduly excludes the possibility of local 'traditional' views on the witch eluding the fieldworker studying urban, cosmopolitan settings. The theory is immune to this possibility precisely because it has become controversial to state that these settings are more likely to exhibit varieties of modernity, or to surmise that they are epistemologically less challenging than a rural network of initiated healers (and therefore are currently more favoured by researchers due to increased time-constraints). It seems that a possibility inhering our very discipline's methodology, of openness to radical cultural difference, has been tabooed, just at a time when the methodological advances of the last decades have made such difference more accessible than in Evans-Pritchard's days.

To reverse the tide of globalist thought, I propose to narrow down our notions of magic and modernity, so that, respectively, there can be things non-magical and modernities can be the plural of something (and consequently the opposite of something) formerly known as tradition. This should provide a more solid basis for theorizing. Furthermore, it is only by defining modernity and witchcraft distinctively that we can fully register the claim of this book: modern reason and the construction of the witch display the same structure of experience. Witchcraft is not a response to modernity, nor itself a form of modernity. Modernity specializes in an aspect of witchcraft.

A large chunk of the cited literature can be summed up as operating on the following syllogism: witchcraft is enchantment, and modernity enchants; hence the modernity of witchcraft. This analysis could not have been more wrong. Firstly, modernity, as an epistemology, does disenchant. Secondly, the idea of the witch stems from disenchantment too. It is magic that enchants, which is something else. 'The modernity of witchcraft' thesis assembles a cluster of associations, which comprehensive and in-depth ethnography could have disentangled.

The first thing that needs disentangling is the idea of magic being illicit. Failing to properly distinguish the user of magic, or the sorcerer, from the witch is one of the most recurrent traits of the witchcraft literature since the Comaroffs (1993) until Harry West's (2007) recent contribution. As Ranger (2007) critically notes, the popular catch-all 'the occult' jumbles together anything from white and black magic to child witches and even ritual (which to some can seem occult for not resembling Catholic liturgy). The use of magic is not illicit in Sukuma culture, despite its concealment and despite national policies of discouragement. Traders and lovers regularly use potions of seduction (*samba*). A cautious household head protects the family with black magic called *lukago*, to which the intruder, thus witch, will succumb.

Differences within Africa today are sharper than those between Africa and Europe. By classifying all African societies as 'modernities' we fail to account for the tension between Sukuma village communities and highly Christianized centres where magic is abjured and a crucial distinction has eroded, namely that between the protective use of black magic and a magical attack that is unsolicited. The latter attack, for no reason except envy, has the marks of the witch, called *bulogi*, literally 'witch-ness', for which we may use the term 'witchcraft'. Although it comprises poison and ingredients of 'access' just like magic, its moral tenor is very different from magic. While I use the words sorcery and magic interchangeably, I follow Kapferer (1997: 12; 2003) in pursuing the idea behind Evans-Pritchard's distinction between sorcery and witchcraft, between respectively conscious use of magic and unconscious malicious effect. If we broaden the concepts, we can make sense of the bulk of ethnographic data worldwide where the (secret, despicable) 'witchcraft' within the kin group is oppositely valued to the 'sorcery' of kings, great practitioners, cults and warriors (public, ludic if often lethal). But it is also true that, like Sukuma, many cultures do not make the terminological difference (unlike Evans-Pritchard's Azande) nor know of an unconscious evil attack. What then is the difference between witchcraft and sorcery (or magic) about? I argue that they stand not for two practices but for two structures or frames of experience, disenchantment and enchantment. They contrast the powerless state of the bewitched with the empowered state of users of magic.

The witch is despised. Yet, how could magic be illicit if the mark of initiation among Sukuma is the possession of magical recipes and the knowledge of more than forty plants and magical ingredients? Magic is associated with knowledge and with membership in a society, which partakes of the larger social system and the informal medico-political network. The fixed association of magic with crime is typical of places without public initiatory traditions. Stories can sometimes be heard of a trader performing the criminal act of sacrificing his child's mental capabilities in return for success, but these are stories falling outside the public initiatory context. I do not discount the idea that stories and rumours, just like beliefs, can lead a life of their own and after a while motivate actions by healers and clients, but this insight is not the major contribution I would reserve for anthropology. Our contribution consists in finding the structures behind those diverse and changing beliefs. For that purpose ethnographic fieldwork moves from the discourse on witchcraft – stories told to an interviewer – to observation of situations of creative practice when witches come into being and the bewitched want treatment.

Globalist approaches lose sight of the experiential processes their own social analysis presupposes, and of the differences that locally matter such as that between magic and witchcraft. This results in the loss of an important reflective and creative dimension in their analysis of culture. Consider the social explanation of witchcraft: modernity gives rise to inequalities, winners and losers, that locally necessitate occult explanations in which the winners are suspected of using magic and the losers are suspected of holding grudges and are therefore labelled as witches. About the losers as suspects, Jean and John Comaroff (1993) argue along with a host of historians that in late medieval Europe the witch was modernity's 'prototypical malcontent', such as an elderly woman representing traditions that obstructed the upcoming merchants' capitalist aspirations. This hypothesis is attractive, however in the end indicative of the more general problem these studies run into. The data are correct but their interpretation hinges on a reality of experiential structures left implicit. To clarify: the woman herself need not be malcontent; she is experienced as such by others. It is they who bring her into being as a witch. The authors make abstraction of the subject's presumptive process, an experiential process, and so place the witch's spell on a par with a fortune-seeker's use of magic. Together they would form the category of malcontents. There is a reason why the thesis on witchcraft as a riposte to the excesses of modern capitalism refuses to make explicit the experiential process this riposte to crisis supposes. The 'modernity of witchcraft' thesis retains an essentialist approach to culture. Socialized cultural patterns (beliefs) predict responses to modernity, which differ between the content and malcontent. What about the beliefs, down to their detailed content, every time again arising from and being shaped by the situation, rather than applying old patterns? Beliefs arise from a situation we can share, not from a cultural source secluded from us. How else could we, as outsiders, recognize these processes, or at least their outcome within a larger field of human possibilities? Here we have it, the result of twenty years of epistemological silence: an anthropological observer invisible and transcendent to the events would be registering the actions and reactions of others programmed by their culture. This view is in accordance with Bourdieu's praxiology and the wider trend since the 1990s of globalisation studies concentrating on the social life of things, their flows and influences, eventually banking on a historicism whose explanatory model revolves around the objectivist chimera of one atom propelling another.

If we consider socio-experiential frames in actions and beliefs, we have more chance of eliciting cross-cultural affinities that could not be derived from observing the practice or hearing the belief. Without the experiential dimension, we would classify magic and witchcraft together under the occult. Subsequently, from the observation that each modernity has its concept of evil and that commodity capitalism is rarely part of this concept, and that magic is not illicit, we would have to reject Taussig's association between people's recourse to magic and their implicit critique of commoditization (Englund 1996; Geschiere 1997). However, once we see the experiential opposition between the sorcerers we all are and the witch, it shows that Taussig's theory, while perhaps failing to account for Sukuma having no misgivings about commodity capitalism, certainly captures their negative connotation of commoditization, because witch construction resembles its logic whereas magic does the opposite.

The owner of a large herd of cattle with a prosperous family will generally be deemed an expert in magic, not a despicable witch. His success may arouse envy and rumours about selfishness (*budoshi*), but the general disapproval of *bulogi*, the unsolicited attack out of envy, indicates that what Sukuma villagers really despise is precisely the moralism of imposing restraint – a modest life style and more charity, for example – on the successful accumulators, on the 'winners' of the competition in magic. So, for the Sukuma I worked with there was nothing immoral about the market or commodity exchange or even individualist accumulation. What they despised in the witch is a worldview, an attitude to life or what I have called an experiential structure. To outsiders, the difference between the witch and the user of magic (exemplified in the dancer; see Chapter 3) may be a matter of nuance, but to Sukuma it is crucial. It dawned upon me after my initiation into the society of elders, *bunamhala*, where much emphasis is put on magical knowledge and novices are trained into differentiating tenors of experience. In a time when some of the anthropological literature has come to view the use of magic as symptomatic of, and as reactive to, capitalist pressures, it is important to stress that a certain aspect of modern capitalism is actually in line with an aspect of magic, namely the adoption of special knowledge and technology in a competition for power, with individual inequalities preceding and arising from that competition (although somewhat balanced by clan belonging). Magical knowledge and ingredients are not for free. A Sukuma pays for initiation. Once initiated, one climbs in formal status by treating the other members to beer and food. Those with a food surplus have an advantage. But as I argued, in another aspect magic fundamentally differs from modern capitalism, for the user of magic admits to need 'access', *shingila*, and accepts its uncertainty (while moderns more likely reject the idea of access, or subsume it under religion, and claim to 'live with contingency' but nevertheless strive for certainty). Initiation itself can be understood as an exercise in experientially differentiating the user of magic and the witch. Victor Turner (1967) famously described the liminal phase of initiation rituals, a moment of anti-structure when the social order is inverted and novices undergo an emotional ordeal that prepares them for the bodily inculcation of norms. During the *ihane* ritual discussed in chapter 3 (wherein I participated) this moment of apparent anti-structure actually initiated the novices into other structures of experience than the normative one. During the ordeal we explored the limits of sacrificial logic and what the unfathomable depths of anxiety can drive people to, and indirectly what witches do: their perverting of social exchange. In the liminality of ritual, structures emerged that revolved around the border, *limen*, between magic and witchcraft. At the height of creativity, when the society's teachers share their knowledge with the novices in a series of what seemed to be ad hoc inventions, one *bunamhala* teacher hung a heavy rock around our necks and whispered in our ear *sengi*, the word for father's sister, a highly charged action verging on witch construction (see Chapter 5). The distinction between a witch and a user of magic could also get hold of the participant's experience more surreptitiously, as the ritual positively filled in what a magical attitude to life is about, and to illustrate this, gift and sacrifice alternated throughout the rituals (cf. Chapter 3). At the risk of violating an unspoken code among fieldworkers, I cannot bracket the value of my initiation. It offered a standard for comprehending witchcraft and for distinguishing it from magic. I learned something epistemological and experiential that, to my knowledge, has remained absent in the massive field of witchcraft studies – too conspicuously to not have a cultural reason.

It has been claimed that modernity enchants and therefore reinforces witchcraft beliefs. The claim is misleading because, as I have just argued, it covers up the contrast with magic, as well as the disenchantment the witch stands for. If witches remind us of modernity, it is because of the pure reason in their construction. But from the other side of the equation the thesis is misleading too, because it underestimates the disenchanting force that is modernity.

Contemporary analyses of witchcraft have been defending the plurality of 'modernities' to the point of neglecting what modernities are the plural of. Modernity, in the singular, does stand for something severely disenchanting, I contend. The diversity of Christian, Hindu, Islamic and other religious expressions cannot conceal that global communication in economy, media, politics and education is largely dominated by oneness in terms of epistemology, at least if compared to the magical epistemology the reader will be introduced to. About half a century after Tylor's blandly evolutionist separation of magic, religion and science, anthropologists denounced any comparison of the three. Might the general denouncement have been motivated by a problematic agreement with Tylor that magic is the weaker third in the battle raging between religion and science? Tambiah (1990) revived the comparison by treating magic as one 'ordering of reality' next to other orderings, but a plurality does not contradict hierarchy.

The only way to deconstruct it is to investigate the premises it relies on. Then it will appear that once we manage to disentangle witch-constructs from magic, the domain of the so-called occult bifurcates. Witch-constructs have to be associated (qua logic and subjective experience) with the most improbable of the three orderings, the scientist's positivism. It inevitably raises a question in this new era of witchcraft accusations calling for the eradication of witchcraft beliefs: whether positivism is the best way to combat such constructs. Is a neo-colonization of consciousness (following that of the missionaries) the solution, or is it part of the problem? Has that neo-colonization not already begun? School curricula, socio-economic development projects, international and national governments (whether plainly neoliberal or African-style socialist, such as Nyerere's *ujamaa*) share one thing: the request made of 'Sukuma' to be 'realistic', to look at neighbouring populations in Arusha, Bukoba, Kenya and Rwanda, to listen to school teachers, and insert themselves in the new global power structure, to wit, into a hierarchy where they will occupy the lowest rank that provides the system's resources. The longer it takes before Sukuma follow the example of their neighbours, the less chance they will have to climb the global ladder leading to liberation, to the heavens above, which their parents never believed in. Perhaps an extreme example are their neighbours to the west in Rwanda, where 'traditional indigenous belief' has allegedly dropped since colonization to an unreal 0.1 per cent of the population (see chapter 7). It is not that these development projects, and the civil society connected to it, want Sukuma to give up their culture as an 'identity'.[3] They welcome Sukuma music and dance performances and, some day, Sukuma restaurants. No, they want Sukuma to give up their culture as a set of experiential structures, as a gradually developed and (through trial and error) collectively crafted set of perspectives on the world that, because being as human as ours, could question ours. The whole discourse about respect for cultural identity, which anthropology has come to support as a discipline, fits within an active process of globalization, rendering cultures adaptable to an 'open-ended' and 'multiple' modernity, and to the rationality of the Swahili buzz word: *maendeleo*, 'development' as progress. The bottom-line of the development endeavour is that Sukuma must recast their culture as an instance of a poor standard of life and, echoing the colonial view, due to a lack of 'education'. Nobody seems to doubt that the net result of the Western striving for better technology and medical cures is, quite simply, more happiness for all. Nobody seems to doubt that a radical difference between cultures is an outdated idea and an unpleasantly divisive one at that (and that includes anthropologists, urban and rural, cosmopolitan and other). It takes the courage of a Tanzanian hip-hop artist to transcend the opposition between the (neo)colonizers and the subaltern, and recognize the divisions within the latter. In this respect the book will at some stage contrast individual and collective reason, and discuss the recent growth of witch killings in Sukuma villages, and finally make the (admittedly risky) comparison with the genocide that took place some two hundred miles west of these villages.

It would be incorrect to suggest, as I was often told by Tanzanian development workers, that Sukuma refuse to sign themselves up to the global reality of modernity. Rather, and despite its plurality, it is this global reality that has certain common traits which have excluded Sukuma farmers. For example, the colonial introduction of cotton as a cash crop led Sukuma smallholders to unite in a massive cotton cooperative in 1955. The backlash came in the 1970s with the national government's integration of this local initiative through nationalization, meaning centralization, top-down management and regular embezzlement of the revenues. Later on, Nyerere's *ujamaa* villagization programme – which aimed to bring people closer to the dispensary, cotton store and school – did not go down well with Sukuma farmers, for it again promoted central authority and even 'oneness' (*umoja*, a Swahili term) which meant acceptance of not only ethnic identities but, more fundamentally, a disregard of cultural difference. That is, socio-economic interventions were promoted regardless of the local cosmology, itself developed over time and deeply rooted within the natural and social environment, including the climate and the soils, and the ways of life, which suddenly had to deal with something one could term over-socialization. The development projects organized by educated members of Tanzania's 'civil society' were cut from the same cloth, seeing in the Sukuma politico-medical system an enemy of progress. Social scientists currently assisting these projects are not aware that their effort to adapt the projects to the culture only hinders resistance to the model the projects represent. In my experience, Sukuma farmers will not

29

tell them about the sensed pressure, partly because the experiential structure of 'development' operates surreptitiously in its postcolonial guise, and because there is too much ground for misunderstanding to even begin mentioning the pressure. The risk is that the projects pull out. The loss of money in the short term will always seem a greater evil than the unsure effect in the long run of eroding a culture's experiential palette.

# Moral Power (II)

Through case studies of medical treatments, the next chapter gradually introduces the reader to Sukuma epistemologies of healing. We shall not be content with public discourse on the witch's black magic. Stories of the occult heard in the media, the bars, the churches and the streets are definitely one side of the phenomenon, and one of growing influence as other sources of information such as rituals and cults initiating into magic lead a clandestine life. Yet, in concrete situations of therapy, people appear to concentrate on something less patent than someone's use of magical ingredients: the witch's moral power. That is what kills. That is the witchcraft in magic. The grudge, whether or not justified in the victim's eyes, gives the witch access. That access is of a different order to the magical ingredient's uncertain access, *shingila*. The social and experiential situation transforms. The grudge becomes a curse, *ndagu*, perverting the ancestor into an accomplice. The diviner seeks to uncover not only the magical ingredients applied by the witch but also the latter's claim to the victim's life. The witch's moral power draws from the sacrificial dimension, the umbilical tie between subject and group, the very thing that normally feeds people's capacity to live with uncertainty about others (might they be witches?) and about oneself in part (how's my ancestral guide doing?). Sukuma farmers have developed a ritual apparatus to deal with moral power. Had they gone for the radical solution of rejecting the sacrificial altogether, they probably would have resembled more the workers, consumers and believers the modern developers have in mind. But the developers never ask what the price might be of restructuring people's collectively crafted experience of the world. The fairly recent rise of witch killings may be part of the answer.

That is the theory in a nutshell. Throughout the book ethnographic sections will alternate with comparative analysis. Their ultimate argument will be that if the name and concept of the witch died under modernity we cannot also claim that its experiential structure, moral power, did. I dare wager that the lethal claims of moral power surge stronger than before in the world precisely because we got rid of their name, which diviners could make us remember. Consider the driving force of reproach in media, academics and politics. Stronger still, what else but the intense belief in moral power has sustained the cycle of systematic violence since the peak of modernity, leading from Versailles to Auschwitz, from Auschwitz to Israel, from Israel to the Twin Towers, and from there to Iraq? Why can we not expel the evil?

It is premature to go deeper into these matters prior to the ethnography. But to hint at what follows: Sukuma let an unknowable evil, the witch, come to life in oracles so as to subsequently turn the table on the witch in rituals publicly showing how the community and the ancestors side with the victim. Magic and oracle also restore people's experience of a holistic universe. They leave participants with a feeling largely kept unspoken: 'Aren't we all witches?' Then the cycle of deadly claims has little chance of enduring.

Back home it made me wonder whether one can substitute science for divination without in the long run winding up in Western specialties: world war, exploitation, colonization, proselytism. Probably diviners have been responsible for wars in the past, but the benefits I refer to concern the experiential structure stimulated in a culture (from which the invention of divination emanates). Anthropology's silence at this experiential, comparative level has kept a 'hungry' public uninformed about such epistemologies that are not positivist and therefore less likely to translate belief into action, such as witch-killing. Of course, a hindrance is that the issue is intercultural, in the sense of one culture discussing another. It requires something anthropology has barely begun to develop: a comparison of experiential structures at a holistic level integrating the the Westerner's cultural premises. The 'modernity of witchcraft' thesis brackets those premises as it situates witches in postcolonial history. It expects anthropologists to ignore the parallels across history and cultures, and disconnect witches as modernity's malcontents from precolonial witches and from the enduring pattern of moral power. The 'experiential structures' thesis explores the epistemological relations, against our historicist inclination.

The killing of innocent elderly ladies on the basis of suspicions and oracles occurs in Sukuma villages, but is not representative of cultures embracing magical epistemologies. Firstly, this experiential structure can be found in scientific cultures as well, and secondly, the tenor of magical epistemologies by and large is precisely not to take beliefs and oracular visions that literally. The literal interpretation of beliefs has rather been the Western ethnographer's (textualist) bias. The slaying of a witch is not exactly compatible with the use of counter-magic. Execution does not tally with a healthy dose of uncertainty about ancestral spirits and witches. (In the old days execution was the prerogative of the chief, who stood outside the gift system). Nobody, including the diviner, really 'knows'. One is free to consult several diviners and make up one's mind. Witchcraft beliefs thus partake of a dynamic of shifting experiential structures that have been meticulously differentiated over centuries in small communities. The initiation rituals further familiarize adolescents with the use of magic. I will relate this practice to 'peace', *mhola*, literally 'coolness', a word Sukuma use in every greeting and which refers at once to social and personal peace. In comparison we may ask what role is played by modern forms of government, schooling, media and Churches, among others. An epistemological transition is taking place whereby people learn to take beliefs literally as well as desert traditional training in magic. In such a transitional context witchcraft can become a dangerous idea, turning spontaneous surges of aggression into systematic violence. Magic then finally becomes what moderns take it for, if only because of the frame moderns take for granted and unwittingly spread. That modern frame of experience is not new to Sukuma. They have an ancient word for the uninitiated, for the state of novices prior to initiation, left in the forest to themselves without community or ancestors: *busebu*, 'heat', the experiential structure to avoid.

# Magic and Bewitchment: Experiential Structures

The chapters progressively introduce the reader to the Sukuma healer's epistemology. Instead of neatly integrating beliefs in a cosmology, I start from what matters to healers and patients, and relate or oppose this to the reader's epistemology. This shall lead to four structures of experience: magic as relating gift and sacrifice (Chapter 3), the crisis of bewitchment (Chapter 5), healing through divination and exorcism (Chapters 6 and 9) and the escapism of spirit possession (Chapter 8). All four are each other's opposites suggesting a comprehensive (if far from detailed) classification of relations: reciprocity, intrusion, expulsion and subversion. The next chapter brings the reader right into the compound of a female healer, Seele, who treats the affliction of *mayabu*. Through the therapeutic itineraries of her patients, we learn about illness and how magic works. The chapter's ethnography is important for the flow of arguments throughout the text.

The ethnography becomes anthropology, however, in the holistic sense defended above, only after the Sukuma concepts are defined in relation to our own. A century of culturally particularist descriptions in ethnography cannot conceal the recurrence of oppositions underlying Western conceptions of other people's beliefs such as sacred-profane, male-female, day-night, order-wild. As long as we do not map (structure) the terrain of cultural interpretations, our descriptions will fall back on intuitive paths that only look different because of the exotic labels we present them with. Therefore, every bit of ethnography on Sukuma epistemologies of healing will be interpreted through a comparative language, more exactly in terms of the forms of social exchange I introduced earlier. The comparative language will in turn give rise to cross-cultural hypotheses, applied to psychotherapy (Chapter 2), social exchange and moral economies (Chapter 4) and the issue of violence, especially witch killings and genocide (Chapter 7). We will come to conceive of Sukuma culture anthropologically, that is, not as a unique, separate symbolic system for ethnographers to objectify but as a historical stimulation of certain states over others within a set known to the human organism. To apply the two dimensions mentioned earlier, a culture is a people as well as a certain place on the map of meaning; the people is not stuck to any place.

Anyone building a theory on structures of cultural creativity will find witchcraft an ideal point of entry. Ethnographers have known for a long time that there exist patterns in the creation of witches; that there are 'usual suspects' in terms of gender and kinship position (see, e.g., Gluckman 1970; Marwick 1970). The topic has never been fully explored, and over time I have noticed how scholars within the field avoid it. This is understandable, if unfounded (and perhaps illuminating for those wondering why our field is accumulating the taboos). True, since fixed categories of witches mean innocent people die because of cultural beliefs, they invoke what none of us wants: instances that might justify colonial and missionary intervention in non-Western cultures. The purport of my argument, and the reason why I would introduce experiential frames in the study of culture, is that this reasoning abstracts the dynamic of experiential frames accompanying beliefs. What, I ask, is actually happening when the Sukuma healer's patients spontaneously come to suspect the paternal aunt; when they say her motive for killing a nephew is her demand to get back 'the cattle of her lap' (*ng'ombe ja matango gakwe*); when, in an extremely condensed manner, people suggest that she would be entitled to the life of her brother's offspring in return for the sacrifice she made of supporting the gift system by marrying and arriving empty-handed in the husband's clan? The 'bewitched' hereby achieve something of a cosmological reversal. They turn their own culture inside out (which our theories of socialization think impossible – another hurdle to overcome by ethnographers of witchcraft). The bewitched namely reject the traditional distinction between gift and sacrifice. The sacrifice women make is no longer seen as mere duty. Their sacrifice is reinterpreted as a gift, which creates a bottomless debt entitling them to the life of their brothers' children. So, when we look at the sort of witch constructed, we notice a disregard of tradition, a disregard of the most central tenet of magic. That is what we understand by modernity, epistemologically speaking. What emerges in the Sukuma healer's compound is modernity; or, better still, the ever modern. The diviner expels it. The possessed becomes it. That is what this monograph is about.

The upshot of this hypothesis should thoroughly unnerve students of witchcraft. The witchcraft in magic is too modern for us moderns to comprehend. Any epistemological comparison we make is suspect. Now comes the ploy of this book, which is based on a straightforward find. The healer's compound is a place where cultural comparison unfolds before our eyes. The inhabitants shift between the various perspectives that happen to be the protagonists of our debate, including the frame of the ever modern, which, I have just claimed, besets our analyses. Together with the healers, their patients and apprentices, we cross a fence and leave the community's everyday cosmology of magic behind. During the period of apprenticeship, in the objects we handle, in the interactions we engage in, and in the sensations we have, we experience the clash between the rationalist cosmology of the bewitched and the sacrificial cosmology of the healer, and more. We gradually grow into one frame and then into the next. Places or *topoi* may be a better term as the contours of the frames are hazy and a matter of choice in specificity. In our non-Cartesian approach the category of units – such as 'frames', 'structures' and others – matters less than their distinction, their relation. That is of interest to the healer's rituals, plant medicine and group therapy, hence to us, because of what distinctions imply: shifts between the units. A change of place, in a socio-experiential sense, can heal.

The reality of opposite structures, explaining genuine shifts of mood and perception, became visceral to me in the initiatory rites I participated in. For instance, in the *Chwezi* spirit cult the separation between male and female worlds disappears. But when memorial services were held for a deceased leader, another shift took place. Halfway through the sacrifice of the goat representing the deceased, the women were suddenly chased from the house with the words: 'This is a funeral!' The mood of fusion had receded and people sensed during mourning that the village rules were back in order, in this case with regard to sexual separation.

Another example is the sharp discussion I witnessed during a meeting of the *Chwezi* cult when someone proposed not to treat the ones unable to pay the fees. One tall elder stood up and gained approval when protesting in a carrying voice that the money required for treatment should not intervene with the patient's ancestral call. All present sensed the tensions between the experiential frames of therapy, business and the spirit's call. The same social domain, the spirit cult, gave way to three states, which are extendable to other domains of society.

35

The concept of interrelated frames resolves a number of problems troubling the discipline. Until now I have argued that their epistemological and experiential depth challenges dominant *globalism* and *historicism*, and that their plurality overcomes the *moralism* of dichotomous assessment. But there are three more pitfalls avoided, each related to our discipline's linchpin, the culture concept. The first is the substantivist, *atomistic* concept of culture, whereby we imagine groups and their ideas getting into contact, sometimes into conflict or shock, and responding with either resistance to, or appropriation of, the other group's ideas. If one ignores the more universal relations behind cultural ideas, one will naturally be astonished about the presence of magic in modern societies, or of modernity in magical practices. Anthropologists have indeed been successful at illustrating how cultures appropriate new ideas through local structures, a classic example being Melanesian cargo cults (e.g., Lattas 1998). But once the analysis envisages a more general level of structures, such as 'magic' and 'modernity', we must ask whether these structures are culturally unique. By revelling in the fact that our modern institutions produce all kinds of enchantment, including 'magical cognition' (cf. Sörensen 2006), we focus on the ideas or beliefs and set aside the epistemological relations between magic and modernity. That is a recipe for exoticizing both, for exclaiming: 'Look how magical our modernity (still) is!' Case in point are the contributions to Meyer and Pels (2003) showing that modern societies often do not reject but 'incorporate' magical ideas, as well as produce them. Cultures would atomistically consist of ideas that are picked up or collide. In my approach they can be epistemologically related, for instance opposed. Meyer and Pels (ibid.: 16) apply magic and witchcraft interchangeably, and define magic cross-culturally through polythetic elements such as subconscious processes of self-deception and suggestion, explanations of misfortune, and exaggerated optimism. All these elements come close to associating magic with irrationality (for which a cognitivist explanation would be better placed). Contemporary anthropologists of magic overlook the epistemology in its own right, which explains why they are the first generation thinking they could write about magic without having studied traditional healing.

Experiential frames or structures prevent a second common mistake, known as *culturalism*. In-depth interviews with healers, observation in their compounds, and the study of genealogies of death will together indicate that the witch constructed by Sukuma embodies a structurally intrusive figure, an 'outsider within' – such as the aforementioned paternal aunt, or the grandmother, who comes from another clan but controls the inner core of the house. Jackson (1989: 96ff) similarly observed among the Kuranko of Sierra Leone that the witch is 'someone within the household yet in league with enemies without', or like owls: wild yet living in the village. However, my purpose in emphasizing the role of experience in culture is to show that any cultural belief, such as the intruder being a witch, has to be experientially framed otherwise we commit the culturalist error of assuming that somebody could be persecuted as a witch for occupying a structurally intrusive position. It takes a frame first, one radically disenchanting the subject's experience – for example, following grave misfortune, affliction or sustained social stress – before that persecution happens. Figures of crisis are explanatory because they capture the subject's experience, not the other way around. Persecuting people because they are stigmatized is another process altogether.[4]

Besides atomism (or substantivism) and culturalism, the distinction of experiential structures remedies a third tendency of the culture concept: *essentialism*, or the separation of cultures by equating each with an incommensurable 'perspective' or experience of the world. When experiential structures thus coincide with cultures, they lose their point of existence. The advantage of recognizing a structure behind disparate cultures, as Lévi-Strauss (1962) found out, is that it undermines the tendency of othering or exoticizing cultures. The recognition of structures works in both ways. For too long the theoretical debates preoccupying Africanists have operated on the assumption that these debates are impermeable to the African cultures themselves. I show that Sukuma practices have epistemologies, and that we thus may learn *from* Sukuma, rather than just about them, however unlikely this may sound to those who judge a tree by its fruits and think an instance of those fruits to be the poverty and witch-killings for which Sukuma in particular have been targeted in both international and national media. In remarkable contrast to the world philosophies of 'great civilizations' in Asia that inspire Western academics, it seems that social scientists have never known how to really engage with African epistemologies. There have been metaphysical derivations for sure, such as Griaule's (1975) notorious construct claiming to have plumbed the depths of Dogon cosmology. Overcoming Griaule's hermeticism, there have been African philosophers rendering local epistemologies conversant with Western debates and critically wedding both cultural perspectives to global challenges, instead of essentializing 'Africa' (Appiah 1993; Wiredu et al. 2004). But the exercise has not been done in a way that could shake Western epistemology because the terms have remained the latter's. Hountondji (1983) argues that these terms, including the critical view on traditions, are precisely what separate philosophy from African traditional thought, which is misrepresented as 'ethnophilosophy'. Mudimbe (1988) offered the alternative of approaching it as gnosis, a secret initiatory wisdom. I would not want to overplay my hand, and even suggest that this book will make a difference. But each chapter proposes what may have been lacking: an experiential take on gnosis, which implies the double move of laterally connecting the 'philosophies' while going deep enough in the cultural matter. Participation in the practice of divination, in spirit possession and in the invention of medicine can tell us things that words, myths, proverbs, beliefs and cosmological descriptions cannot.

# The Senses in Healing

To sum up, we will come to a surprising insight after distinguishing the use of magic from the construction of witches. The witch arises neither from irrationality, as evolutionist anthropologists had it and contemporary scholarship again insinuates, nor from everyday rationality, by which Evans-Pritchard (1976), Lévi-Strauss (1962) and Horton (1967) thought to respect non-modern practices. Nor does it arise from a-rationality, as suggested by scholars today finding in unconscious desires a way to respect those practices. Rather, it arises from the remaining option, the only one that does not leave modern ideology intact: the witch is constructed from pure reason.

What inventers of healing rites have found out is that bewitchment means a life dominated by an invisible moral power, a life 'reduced' (*ku-geeha*) to the look of others, to use an expression cited later on. Yes, healers speak of witches, spirits, forces and other invisible entities that will convince scientists of the unreliable basis of healing rituals. But anthropologists consider the experiential reality these beings embody. They appreciate how, on a sensory level, the rituals have managed to articulate the victim's opaque experience in social terms that permit ritual intervention. The rituals namely tackle the feeling of powerlessness and guilt by attributing it to a certain perspective on the world, namely one that misses the sacrificial dimension hidden in every gift. Rites of exorcism, divination and spirit possession thus socially reorganize experiences, especially relevant in these parts of Africa where illness and death are frequent and the capacity for self-healing is often the main source of recovery.

This brings us to a final theme: the therapeutic efficacy of magic and ritual. The label of 'traditional religion' has paternalistically shielded them from scientific scrutiny. Yet, Sukuma rituals and magic have always taken place within a context of healing rather than worship. Much of their healing power, as we will see, lies in their recognition of illness and misfortune as a holistic reality connecting various elements, from the social to the sensorial, into an encompassing 'state of the system'. This connectivity accounts for the importance of the senses in ritual and magic. As the interface of mind and body, the senses mediate these states. Healers initiate sensory shifts between these frames, irrespective of the Cartesian divide preoccupying academics. Such ease in crossing the divide is how I comprehend magic. Sensory shifts explain how patients could physically improve due to something seemingly 'symbolic' like magic.

The next and last chapters discuss the treatment of *mayabu*, a condition akin to schizophrenia. As long as we consider meaning to be a non-physical attribute of physical substances, magical remedies will remain incomprehensible to us. Once we discover the verb stressing the activity in the word 'meaning', and read it as 'relating', we may apprehend the materiality of magic. Analogous to clinical synaesthesia (colours generating sounds), magic seems to operate on a synaesthetics that couples certain semantic structures with states of the organism. While cultural sensoria predispose to the coupling of meaning and matter, healers have a knack for further codification of the senses. A patient's insertion into a healer's synaesthetics of turning meaning into matter is part of the healing process.

How to explain the occurrence of witchcraft, divination, magic and spirit possession across the world? Cultural diffusion from a common origin? Our human biology as the common origin? Experiential structures in my view answer the anthropological puzzle by offering the holistic alternative. What we recognize across cultures are not the exact practices of witchcraft, divination and so on (which are never the same) but structures, orderings of the whole. These are not located in origins but in outcomes, namely in our interpretations and representations of the practices. Sahlins (1976) and Geertz (1973), whose concepts of culture largely shaped the discipline as it stands today, were not blind to cross-cultural patterns, but were quick to defend the specificity and autonomy of each culture, lest we resort to biological mechanisms (or today's version: evolved cognitive faculties) as explanations of universal traits. They assumed universality to require causal explanations (which they contrasted in Weberian manner with cultural *interpretations*). Many authors since have seemed to fear the colonization of our subject by the 'other' side, natural science. Yet, the daunted should know that positivist explanations themselves follow from an ordering of reality, which is not an ordering of facts; a fact results from an experience that orders reality. Perhaps they have not fully faced its ramification: the scientist's orderings are made of the same 'stuff' as the healer's orderings. 'Relations' and 'structures' are other words for that stuff.

Anthropology had the great opportunity to step out of the objectivist position and holistically compare meanings and offer an alternative to the mechanistic worldview, something worthy of the collected voices of non-Cartesian epistemologies they had the honour to study. Instead, after rejecting Lévi-Strauss, many chose to imagine a Tower of Babel, a particularism to beat the god of universalism. So it has come that it sounds subversive today to ask the question I shall begin with: why magic works.

# Notes

1.  See also the studies of witchcraft in Melanesia by Kelly (1976) and Knauft (2007).
2.  Adult literacy in Tanzania was estimated at the time of my fieldwork to be a little over 30 per cent (EIU 1998: 18). Most young adults nowadays have had four or more years of schooling, but this is certainly not a Sukuma priority. In the mid 1990s many households informally divided up tasks, including writing.
3.  This is the development priority. However, I have yet to meet a Sukuma farmer who thinks of their culture as an identity to be defended.

# Chapter 2
# Why Magic Works: Systemic Healing

The first time I witnessed the work of 'the shell', *nonga*, was late at night on returning to the compound of my host, the healer Lukundula. As his son and I neared the entrance, we heard the frenzied speech of a woman in great distress. From the cluttered words we discerned fragments in Swahili, 'Jesus is my saviour!' and 'He will punish you!' Swahili, the Tanzanian national language, was not commonly heard in the village, and nor was the name of Jesus. A Landrover stood in the middle of the compound, its engine running. In the headlights a young woman was scowling at two men about to administer medicine. One man poured liquid from a Cola bottle into a small shell that was briefly held to her nose. Everybody waited attentively for what would happen next. Within a minute she fell silent and shuffled to the nearest wall. While bending down to sit, she murmured in Sukuma, her mother tongue: 'Don't you think I'm giving up'.

The woman was the daughter of a high-ranking district officer. The driver left without saying a word, returning next morning to pick her up. This was against the advice of the healer who said she looked like suffering from an affliction known as *mayabu*. She ought to be divined and probably needed stay over at his compound for prolonged treatment. The driver laughed and pointed to how she had improved. Without paying he left: rumours about a district officer paying for traditional medicine were to be avoided at the time, ten years ago. One of the healer's sons shrugged at me: 'He'll be back'.

It struck me that whereas I, as an ethnographer, had developed a defensive attitude regarding Sukuma healers, many of the educated Tanzanian elite did not doubt their skills but regarded the distancing attitude appropriate. Experts in magic were to be denigrated because of their lack of scientific schooling, their magic exploited like pills, reduced to their visible impact. The following case studies will show the elite's reductionism to be misplaced, and so too the ethnographer's defensive attitude. Lukundula's treatment of psychosis does not need to be defended. It can stand scientific scrutiny, albeit on the condition that we appreciate the therapy in all its cultural aspects, which are typically comprehensive, addressing a reality that connects body, mind and social environment.

The argument for a comprehensive approach to healing, known as holism, can hardly be called new. If anything qualifies as a grand narrative of medical anthropology, it is precisely this idea of mind and body unified. Not only is it ethically attractive for bridging the gap between the epistemologies of the anthropologist and the people studied, there is also a scientific logic to it. How else but on the basis of mind-body unity, whereby meaning affects matter, can ritual meanings be thought to actually contribute to healing (Devisch 1993; Csordas 1996)? How else but on this basis can psychotherapy be efficacious (Sternberg 2000; Solms 2004)? In fact, the placebo effect, whose existence no scientist could deny, is predicated on the mind-body unity: belief can foster recovery (Kaptchuk 2002; Moerman 2002). What has remained lacking, though, in the study of the mind-body unity is a language to talk of the range of possible connections across mind and body.

The thoughts we have, their neural connections and the social interactions they are part of are three modes of reality. The systemic connections between these modes may account for the healing effect of one modal intervention – improvement of social interactions stimulates physical recovery, for example. To find out how these modes work together we should not stick to a modal perspective, with each scientific field – biology, psychology, sociology and so on – keeping to its own object. Nor should interdisciplinary studies raise much hope, as these merely add up incompatible methodologies. We must venture into a 'transmodal' perspective, one that cuts across these modes to capture what the modes have in common; what one set of biological, mental and social modes is like at a given moment. In other words, we must let go of the modalities of reality to consider their 'orderings of reality', to use Tambiah's (1990: 152) term. These assess the state of the system from a fairly coherent perspective, and determine how it should be. They are of the order of values. Contrary to the Kantian distinction between the factual and the moral, which deprives values of their factual basis, the values appear grounded as they continue to undergo the test of time socially, physically and mentally. The diviner's expertise, which anthropologists are so fascinated with, lies in differentiating and naming these transmodal organizations we call values. Divinatory diagnosis takes after social commentary in not limiting itself to the client's body but assessing the state of the larger medico-political system. The assessment itself affects the client's physical state. More than a window on the world, diagnosis (re)structures experience. This lends both ethnographic and scientific significance to our option for anthropological holism, as I want to insist here before discussing 'the data'.

A major inspiration for our studying states of the system instead of Cartesian subsystems has been the following. Healers apply the same value of 'cooling' (*ku-poja*) to plants driving out poison as they do to rituals expelling a curse. Another value, that of reciprocity with the outside, is reserved for food intake, but also for words of greeting, weddings and initiation ceremonies. A third, negative, valuation subtends distinct phenomena such as poison, guilt feelings and witchcraft fears. Irrespective of their material or mental modality, these all speak the language of intrusion. A fourth, more ambivalent value is that of spirit possession and hallucinogenic substances. They resemble each other closely in familiarizing people with what appears intrusive at first, although in the one case we are dealing with 'culture' and in the other with 'nature'.

However awkward this may sound at first to academic ears used to set matter and mind apart, it is perfectly feasible to treat plants and rituals as only differing in mode (biological versus social) while being equivalent in the value that codifies both. This is not farfetched. After all, the worlds of the biologist and the sociologist are not actually all that far apart since their theories both depend on language, often on similar metaphors with an experiential tenor (cf. Lakoff and Johnson 1980). Where should we situate these similarities? Wittgensteinian language games and Goffman's social roles cannot help us here, since they limit themselves to a subsystem, namely the social, and denote categories therein. They miss out on the holism and healing dynamic of states cross-cutting mind, body and society. Much of the medical anthropology literature could be reread as an initiation into these states by healers and diviners. Even roughly summarized, the reasoning of healers strikes one as intriguingly subtle and, not coincidentally since they were patients first, as extremely well versed in the grimmest depths of their patients' suffering: if illness itself stands for a certain state of the system, organizing a variety of social, cognitive and biological modes of being in a certain way, then one should endeavour to heal the system by rearranging the modes of being according to another value, or structure, than the one imposed by illness. This chapter is a first step in teasing the structures apart. Chapter 6 will detail the practice of divination.

# Self-healing

Nobody ever told me that Seele could heal schizophrenia. What she treats, my Sukuma friends assured me, is an affliction called *mayabu*. How to translate *mayabu*? The ethnographer relies on the local classification first. The term is derived from the verb *ku-yabuka*, 'to scream and act uncontrollably'. The most manifest symptom of *mayabu* is uncontrolled speech punctuated with violent outbursts. From the recognizable fragments of speech as well as the contorted bodily expressions of the sufferer one may conclude that the dominant emotion is profound anxiety. What this anxiety might be about is of less concern to medical doctors than the fact of patients distorting their picture of reality. In contrast, healers consider the content of the patient's fears, using a number of techniques, including divination.

One feature of *mayabu* is that its aetiology concerns witchcraft. Unlike healers in town, those in the village do not have a list advertising the illnesses they treat hanging outside the entrance to their compound. The reason is the pivotal role of the oracle. What may look like bewitchment can after divination turn out to be something else, such as an ancestor's request for their descendant to enter a spirit cult. Therapy involves, to a large extent, making sense of the affliction by discussing and (re)constructing the person's life. Patients and their relatives consult several oracles. Emphasis is less on the label of illness and corresponding remedy than on the deeper cause which patients and relatives help the diviner to determine by verifying intricate emotions and histories of social conflict.

*Mayabu* represents the pinnacle of bewitchment, of betrayed social expectations and possible guilt. Sukuma oppose it to *lusalo*, which is considered incurable but less severe, its symptoms resembling epileptic attacks that reportedly depend on the lunar cycle. Both afflictions are distinguished from *saji*, or 'plain madness', affecting a category of people dwelling the streets and markets in rugs, mostly keeping to themselves. The local classification does not oppose mental to physical disorder. It rather places emphasis on the behavioural, in this case on uncontrolled speech. Medical anthropologists may be tempted to detect in *mayabu* a 'culture-bound syndrome'. Might a speech-related affliction not be telling of Sukuma society, where oratory is so highly valued? By the end of this chapter, when we will have sufficiently appreciated the systemic side of illness, we will drop the idea of culture-bound syndromes strictly defined.

Other behavioural disorders concern a period of confusion, typically following severe malarial attacks, for which Sukuma use the term *nzoka ya ntwe*, 'snake of the head' (*degedege*, in Swahili). The 'snake' inside the head, which refers to the brain, is said to 'shake' during fever. Similar impediments on one's behaviour, hence social functioning, can be found among spirit-induced afflictions such as the *majini* curse from the Swahili coast in the east (derived from the Arabic *djinn*) and the mediumistic call of the *Chwezi* cult from the area in the west bordering Uganda and Congo.

No study has been done yet on *mayabu*. The healers I worked with since 1995 claim that *mayabu* is steadily on the rise. I cannot back up this claim with figures on its occurrence among Sukuma or on its prognosis. Local treatment consists in combining pharmacological and socio-interactive elements within a therapy management group supervised by a traditional healer. During one to two years on average the patients live together with others similarly afflicted at the healer's compound, are initiated at their own pace as an assistant healer, and eventually become classificatory children of that healer. The patient returns home as an initiated (but not necessarily professional) healer. Failure to reintegrate the patient into society is rare (I estimate it at about one out of seven patients in the medical compounds where I worked). Successful reintegration may be partly attributed to the polycentric character of Sukuma villages, which limits social stigmatization by granting much autonomy to the extended family. It may also be attributed to the self-reliance of farmers, which less readily exposes mental disorder than for instance commercial interactions might. But the wider socio-cultural order is not enough to explain the apparently good prognosis. Patients regain strength and zest for life before they return home.

Some hospital nurses in Mwanza Region are aware of this success and have begun to clandestinely refer patients with *mayabu* symptoms to traditional experts. One of the main healers referred to is Seele, with whom I have regularly worked over the past ten years. She has seen the number of *mayabu* patients she treats rise from seven in 2003 to thirty in 2007. The bulk of her knowledge comes from her father Lukundula, who was my host and adopted father during my first fieldwork from 1995 to 1997. To introduce Seele's approach I explore four case studies of patients situated at different points of the therapeutic course.

# The Case of Lemi

For many years I hesitated to classify *mayabu* in terms familiar to Western psychopathology. Even though most therapies were a mixture of transmitted knowledge and an individual healer's inventive adaptations to new afflictions, I tended to treat the therapies as ancient cult traditions. So I wondered how we could compare African traditions with Western concepts such as schizophrenia. Should we not consider these traditions as religious instead of medical? Could healers be of any relevance to medical doctors? Were healers and their rituals not better off with the modern segregation of science and religion, by being categorized under the latter and shielded from the former's scrutiny? It is only as I got to know Lemi and his mother in 2007 that I could no longer ignore the resemblance between this illness, which for many Sukuma represents the pinnacle of bewitchment, and a mental disorder famous in the West, schizophrenia, which our doctors have not find a cure for. I have chosen to begin this study of witchcraft with this resemblance to underline the fact that in terms of the epistemological comparison envisaged by this book I cannot insulate African cultures from the rest of the world. Most of all, I want to show that our paternalistic apprehensions about African knowledge are unfounded. Rather, a two-way exchange might rewardingly alter our Western, apparently limited, understanding of this notorious disorder.

Lemi[1] had been in Seele's care for only two weeks when I met him for the first time. I said things to him but cannot claim we ever spoke. All day long he would engage in activities expressing great distress, his moaning and lamenting progressively growing into ranting and loud screaming, then decreasing again for a while, usually after taking the 'shell' medicine described at the beginning of this chapter. From the tree to which he was tied during his outbursts, from which he could move by about a metre, he would yell and curse at passersby. Additionally, he would scream in agony, laugh chokingly, undress himself, make obscene gestures, cover himself in earth, and lay still in contorted expressions. It did not look different from psychotic episodes recorded anywhere else in the world.

Like other patients in the first phase of treatment, he had his ankles chained together to prevent him from running off or attacking others. The chains (*mnororo*) allowed patients to shuffle slowly between various areas in the healer's compound for washing, medicine-intake, sleeping, eating, cooking and other household activities they participated in according to capacity. Over half of the patients are engaged in this peculiar pattern of spatial movements. The resulting sight of a compound bustling in slow motion starkly contrasts with the sound of the one or two newcomers screaming in agony, often day and night. I wondered how Seele could stand it for twenty years on end. Sukuma do not have a word for holiday.

Seele in principle does not isolate those screaming. On the contrary, Lemi's tree stood in the centre of the compound. In the heat of the day when everyone was resting or lying down under the large tree he would still look down upon us majestically, with risen chest repeating things like 'They won't get me' and 'I am Jesus'. When throwing pebbles or sticks at people, he would be admonished or hit. But nobody thought of isolating him from the compound's public life. Healers and fellow patients were shocked to hear from me that this would be true in my own country. The group's togetherness seems to them essential for recovery: Lemi will in the end become himself again and return to his village; hence he should recover in a social setting such as this, whatever state he might be in now.

Moreover, inhabitants told me that they could live with the noise because each of them had gone through this yelling period. In the yelling they did not see the person at work but the witch who was doing this to him. The idea of witchcraft introduces a split between the affliction and the person, which precludes social stigma for the patients and will, for still other reasons, turn out to serve the healing process. None of the patients I talked to could fully explain their yelling periods. Some speculated that the screams accompanied the patient's desperate warding off of aggressors invisible to others. One former patient guessed their screams were reactions to a 'film played in the head'. Another patient, still in the early phase of treatment and regularly experiencing these episodes, objected to the film hypothesis and said that at the moment of the episode itself he is unaware, only afterwards realizing what he has done. Everyone agreed that awareness of one's condition announces the beginning of recovery. That is when one begins to comprehend the reason for one's stay at Seele's place. Coming to one's senses indicates that the witch's spell is losing its power. At that stage, they added, patients will not complain about the chains which outsiders might find a shocking sight. As we will see, the locking and unlocking of the chains may also have a therapeutic function.

Lemi's attitude always changed dramatically in the presence of his mother, to whom he replied in obedient tone. As is common for care-givers, she lived together with him in the hut in Seele's compound. She washed him at the tree and gave him food there. She admonished, even hit him if he became a danger to others. One afternoon she came to sit down with me and my collaborator Paulo, and recounted his case.

Lemi is the fourth of seven children. The illness started suddenly, a month ago, when he returned from work late at night and woke her up for food. He looked troubled. She heard him cry while he was eating: 'My uncle, my grandfather, why do you want to kill me? How have I wronged you?' Lemi had just started up a business as a street vendor after he had worked in the second-hand clothing (*mitumba*) trade for the aforementioned uncle and grandfather (respectively the brother and paternal uncle of his mother). The clothing business had meant a sudden step up the ladder. An outsider may read between the lines that, if not jealous, the uncle and grandfather might have suspected him of holding back some of his takings.

That night the mother saw his condition deteriorate rapidly. Over the following days he was taken to one diviner after the next. All oracles pointed to witchcraft, but they also comforted him that the ancestral guide would not let him die. A magical combat was going on, of which the anxiety expressed in his state of *mayabu* was the outcome. One of the healers thought he could rid Lemi of his curse, but his ritual expulsion did not work. So Lemi was sent to the dispensary in Mbarika, on the assumption that the oracles were wrong and the disorder followed a common malarial attack. After one day in hospital he got worse. That is when his father told him and his mother about Seele's expertise in Wanzamiso, some fifty kilometres away.

Seele's oracle confirmed the other healers' suggestions on the involvement of witchcraft. As for the witch's identity, it is interesting to note that Lemi's reference to his uncle and grandfather was not taken as conclusive. I was told that the witch's magic may be programmed to make Lemi scream those words and fool the hearer into suspecting innocent people. Lemi's mother confided to us that she rather suspected the grandfather's second wife who had been chased from the village in an earlier case of witchcraft. Her revenge would be to hurt her husband's grandson and falsely implicate her former husband.

## Counter-magic and the Shell

For Seele the oracle is important for deciding on treatment. The botanical treatment of *mayabu* consists of two types of concoction, 'hot water' and 'the shell'. Twice a day at sunrise and sunset, the drums are sounded to convoke patients at the centre of the compound. There in the space between the healer's hut and the ancestral altars the pots of the first medicine are waiting. Residents close to terminating their therapy assist in administering the medicine to newcomers such as Lemi. Afterwards they take their own dose. The first medicine seeks 'to descend the poison' (*kwicha ubusungu*). The slightly bitter powder of pounded roots is mixed with hot water and drank slowly from a cup. The purpose is counter-magic: to 'chase' (*kupela*) the poison from head and heart down to the stomach and out again. The witch's attack entered the body after ingestion of poisoned food or drink or after stepping on a magical 'trap', *mitego*. The roots are combined with a symbolic additive (*shingila*, mentioned in the introduction) that represents the medicine's purpose such as a tiny piece of a broom. The idea is to clean the stomach, physically. The mixture may cause diarrhoea in the first months.

Patients describe the taste of the first medicine as neutral, though slightly bitter. They contrast this with the sensorial effect of the second medicine, for which they move from the first location. They receive it in the space behind the healer's hut and alongside the cattle-pen, close to the rubbish heap. The medicine is called *nonga*, 'the shell', because of the snail's shell from which the liquid is poured into the patient's nostrils. The medicine's container is a fizzy-drink bottle hanging out in the sun on Lukundula's ancestral altars. It comes in two versions: an old Coca-Cola bottle contains the strong version that patients take at the beginning of therapy, while an old Fanta bottle contains the less concentrated version for patients who no longer suffer from logorrhoea or violent episodes. The purpose of *nonga* is to 'settle the mind', *kubeja masala*.[2] It will be useful to discuss some of its ingredients later on to illustrate the value of the systemic approach.

The *nonga* sensation is perplexingly sharp. The liquid and its effect are sensed to travel from the nose to the back of the head, ending in the neck, after which users feel nauseous and may spit. Newcomers react with horror and usually struggle, and so have to be held by assistants. Regular users on the contrary keep their neck backwards for a while and slightly shake their chin to give *nonga* full play. When I probed a young man about his asking for a second dose, he replied: 'I was changing again this afternoon, remember?' I recalled that he had asked me for money that afternoon, with a stern anguished look. After I refused, he went inside his hut, holding behind his back a spoke from the wheel of a bicycle another patient was mending nearby. It surprised me that the others trusted him enough to let him take the spoke.

Minimal interference seems to be the key, as if healing consists not in producing a cure but in taking away the obstruction to the natural process of self-healing. The two medicines – 'descending the poison' and 'settling the mind' – seek to undo the witch's interference and physical impediment respectively. A common term in Sukuma rituals is *tupone*, 'let us ripen', as the natural state of the world. The expulsion of evil intervention attempts to end an obstruction to the natural process. Trust in the medicine, in self-healing and in the group's presence does seem to pay off, as I observed the day I left after my last visit. After a month Lemi not only yelled less but became responsive while yelling. That morning he had synchronized his screams to the ceaseless singing of a new patient. The contest and tonal exchange between the two patients caused much hilarity among all residents. It was a sign that Lemi was on the way to recovery.

## The Systemic Value of Plants

The uncontrolled speech of *mayabu* can take various forms. Alma is a petite elderly lady, who had recently been brought to Seele's compound by her family. She told me not to understand why she was here and what the chains were for. Her only illness, she said, was pain in the lower abdomen. However, for several years she had been roaming out in the bush, only coming home once in a while to eat. She spoke very silently but in a continuous stream, sometimes listening to my questions, then responding with much detail. Slow gestures mimicked her bodily positions from significant situations she recollected, sometimes related to her therapies in the past. As she talked in a flow of often disconnected phrases she would illustrate her descriptions by sitting against a wall, standing up, turning her back on me, or mimicking eating. Paulo remarked afterwards that she had not reached the phase of awareness of bewitchment other patients referred to. Not that the idea was that she would have to. From Alma's account we learned that she had gone through much hardship. As a young woman she was treated for infertility, then after a long while she bore a son. About eight years ago he had passed away, aged nineteen. We wondered if she would ever recover from the blow. Not everyone returns home healed from Seele's place. But what kept her going seemed to be the medicinal plants she took daily. The plants and the bit of food she accepted were her remaining connection with the world.

Plants are remarkable things. They affect people often unnoticeably with their smell or visual presence. As Stoller (1989) and Howes (2003) have argued, sensory input alters the general mood more than ethnographers often realize. In retrospect I wonder why it took me so long to acknowledge the role of plants in Sukuma culture. The Cartesian blind spot of the anthropologist is the matter itself of the plant. As important as the professed meaning is its multi-sensorial impact. Attention for the symbolic obscures it. My initial 'pharmacophobia' if you will is all the more astonishing given the knowledge I had acquired since my initiation into the local society of elders about forty plants occupying a central place. The 'king' (*ntemi*) of every initiatory society is a particular plant, unknown to the uninitiated. Half a year later, during my training for the *Chwezi* cult for spirit mediums, I learned about more medicinal plants and other magical ingredients; I inhaled and drank them, and felt them on my skin.

We may begin to comprehend the importance of plants in magic if we consider their connective role within the larger medico-political system. My Sukuma friends talked about medicinal knowledge and consumed magical concoctions, and wore protective amulets. In a virtually uninterrupted circuit the multi-sensorial exchange with the social and natural environment continued as they ate from the same plate of food and drank beer from a cup shared at night, held hands in the morning to greet each other, and sweated together in the fields, singing in close harmony, then breaking up for lunch. This daily circuit was tied in with the larger interregional dynamic of medicinal exchange, via personal contacts at weekly village markets as well as expanding intra- and inter-clan networks of knowledge. In the dry season some Sukuma travel to the Great Lakes in the west (*Ng'weli*) from where new and potent black magic is said to come and thus recipes have to be bought for the protection of the household. For good fortune in cultivation or trade they visit diviners in the east toward the Great Rift Valley, 'where our ancestors obtained the skill to divine', or they travel and come back from the Swahili towns along the Indian Ocean, where remedies against Arabic spirits (*majini*) can be had. Power and healing become inseparable in an intricate politico-medical network in which healers have informal authority, initiated patients sometimes become community leaders, and where authority figures conversely hold power that is endowed with ritual expertise. In the voyages of medicinal plants the ethnographer unwittingly records some of the ongoing history of the world's first global economy which, from the tenth century, extended from north Tanzania and the Great Lakes to Swahili-speaking East Africa and its monsoon-led connections with the islands of the Indian Ocean and the coasts of the Arabian peninsula and India (see Mitchell 2005). What began as territorial connectivity has – via larger markets, imports, pharmaceutical shops, tourism, the Internet, satellite TV, anthropological research and further migration – obtained a non-territorial and often virtual but no less systemic quality, with extensions to European, Indian and Chinese cities.

Sukuma magic travels across East Africa and beyond to come back altered, carrying with it both the stresses and benefits from the larger system. *Mayabu* affects both men and women, although predominantly young men. A high proportion of them are young traders like Lemi who suddenly become successful and fear reproach or envy within the network of close relatives. While psychiatrists are increasingly inspired by medical anthropologists writing on the social and familial roots of illness and recovery (Lopez and Guarnaccia 2000), they should look into postcolonial studies as well, which reveal the macro-political dimension of affliction: Lemi and several other patients (including the young man with the bicycle wheel spoke) embody the often ambivalent response of farmers to profit-making under modernity and capitalism. What by now deserves the name 'modernity stress' has been observed the world over (Taussig 1980; Shipton 1989; Pred and Watts 1992). The affliction reflects the larger system. The first *mayabu* patient I spoke to, in the first Sukuma healer's compound I stayed in, was a young man who earned a living by digging for diamonds in Mabuki. Every time he was lucky he spent all the money he earned on treating his friends to drinks and gifts. Soon he exhibited the symptoms of *mayabu* and was sent by his family to the healer Solile in Iteja, where I found him after a second relapse. It seems that throughout the cultural system – from the harsh milieu of gold and diamond miners, in the gangsta hip-hop music heard on the radio, to cosmopolitan business – lurks a pathogenic code: a rigid logic of debt and credit whereby nothing – not even love or respect – is gained without paying for it. The communicative system of these young traders and miners seems stuck in a code of transaction, of 'tit for tat', with no relief or mediation by the values they knew in the village such as kinship. There is no ancestral spirit carrying part of the responsibility for these young people's failure or success. The pressure from this code of transaction increases as its particular structure of experience extends from the further corners of the cultural system such as Western and Indian capitalist markets that are regarded by some adolescents as the real centres, where values are decided. Merciless magic is supposed to come from the Great Lakes in the west. Traders presume their competitors to use magic enhanced with the efficacy of the larger system's foreign technology.

Two important elements come to light about magic as well as about affliction: the systemic nature of the environment in which both operate, and the fact of this system being in a certain state. *Mayabu* seems likely in a socio-economic system discouraging any other frame than that of unmediated transaction, such as that of the miner's find resulting in cash or no cash. This intriguingly reminds us of Gregory Bateson's (1990) take on a condition still largely defying Western science and biomedicine, and perhaps therefore arousing the interest of anthropologists: schizophrenia. Bateson (1972) described schizophrenia as someone's tendency to take words literally due to incapacity of dealing with meta-communicative frames. Hallucinatory episodes might be spontaneous attempts of the patient to get some multiplicity back into perception. Something similar will account for the therapeutic effect of spirit possession in the *Chwezi* cult, where novices learn to ritually play on experiential structures (see Chapter 8). The intriguing suggestion, which I would like to further substantiate, is that scientific methodology cannot penetrate the mysteries of the schizophrenic state because it resembles that state. While science is good at labelling the disorder, it cannot tell us what is wrong with it because its mechanistic methodology presuming univocality cannot accept as normal the semantic multiplicity of human experience. Magic, on the contrary, takes the multiplicity of states into account and transforms these.

Confronted with its low success rate, the Western science of psychiatry has become increasingly aware of the failure of psychological models in capturing the systemic reality of mental disorder. The reaction, however, has not been to venture into transmodal analysis, but to add up the modal perspectives; that is, to engage in interdisciplinary research. Psychiatrists thus acknowledge the 'bio-psycho-social' disruption that schizophrenia is, in degrees variable over time, and whose complexity calls for a comprehensive approach such as general systems theory (Peer et al. 2007). Strauss (1989) earlier described the vicious cycle between person and environment whereby feedback loops and compensatory reactions escalate. Hallucinatory experiences originating in the body's homeostatic attempts to canalize stress can be accompanied with certain acts of speech that provoke in the social environment culturally mediated reactions of anxiety, and these in turn aggravate the patient's condition of stress. In other words, 'systemic' implies that a small temporary deficit in immunity may suffice to diminish the patient's contribution to an already precariously balanced household economy and labour force, hence may compel other household members to raise their efforts, eventually straining social relations that were until then peaceful. Macro-social processes undermining traditional norms of kinship and clan alliance may facilitate fission, further depriving the patient from means of relief.

The good news about the systemic nature of illness is that its remedy too can operate systemically, so that a relatively small intervention through a medicinal plant may stimulate recovery across the system. Seele's plants settling the mind and expelling the poison from the body are explicit about the experiential shift of expulsion they intend. There are no guarantees like mechanistic interventions limited to a subsystem. In magic, the way to affect the system is to adopt one value in all modes, from the bodily to the social. For example, one of the five main ingredients of *nonga* medicine is the root of a thorny bush called *busisi*. In combination with saliva, this kind of caper plant, known to pharmacologists as *Capparis fascicularis*, has a significant immuno-stimulant effect and actually calms the brain's dopamine system, which is known to be hyperactive in schizophrenia (Rivera et al. 2003). The *busisi* plant tunes into a homeostatic disturbance and responds to it, just as Seele's rituals and house rules do.

The 'system therapy' Bateson co-founded in the 1960s parallels recent cognitive behavioural therapy (CBT) mostly resorted to in the treatment of 'mental disorders'. The non-Cartesian approach of CBT posits that just as the plant's chemical substances influence thoughts by calming dopamine activity in the brain, so can thoughts (mind) positively rewire the brain (matter) of a patient (see Birchwood and Trower 2006). System therapy and CBT thus concur that schizophrenic patients are stuck in experiential structures they have to get out of. This view does not fundamentally disagree with another classic theory. Psychoanalysis – both Freudian and Lacanian – attributes schizophrenia to the absence of 'a third', somewhat solemnly called the Law of the Father, namely an authority acting as mediator (on top of the mother's input) and from which children deduce that words need not always be believed or taken literally (see Lacan 1973). Love (gratuitous) and desire (earning respect) are two things, sometimes coinciding and sometimes not. In brief, Bateson,

Freud, Lacan, CBT and the Sukuma practitioner all seem to agree on one thing: the importance of experiential shifts.

Inability to shift perspective is a state of rigidity. The concept of states seems therapeutically more sound than a label of disease, such as schizophrenia or *mayabu*, which medicalizes and stigmatizes the condition. The Sukuma idiom of witchcraft refers to an external cause and a state. It is no surprise that of all the psychiatric approaches mentioned, Sukuma magic is most explicit about what the shifts are like. Scientists prefer to keep the values embraced implicit; the label of schizophrenia eclipses psychiatry's values. That is where we might learn from Sukuma. CBT teaches patients suffering from spells of paranoia or from compulsive thoughts to shift their attention to another activity like weeding, or to note the thoughts down when they pop up, or to replace them by positive thoughts (Schwartz 2002). These are ways to tackle a system stuck in a self-destructive state. But surely, not just any diversion of attention does the trick. Weeding may be a good way to shift the patient's attention, but looking at one's watch may exacerbate the condition. There must be some codification, some values at work which inform decisions about what cultural content in a certain context is therapeutic and what is not. Values go beyond the one mode of reality that we as social scientists are supposed to specialize in. Sukuma healers define the transmodal state of *mayabu* through the concept of *ndagu*, a spell, which qualifies a certain combination of bodily, mental and social elements as cursed.

## *Ndagu* Spells: The Transmodal Approach

Before continuing with the case studies, which illustrate the transmodal reality of *ndagu*, I want to summarize Seele's multimodal approach. She combines plants, group therapy and behavioural measures. Ingesting *nonga* from the shell to 'settle the mind' is useless without a therapy group conducive to self-healing. The approach is systemic. It tallies well with the non-Cartesian insight that beneficial effects in one part of the system will positively contaminate the rest because of connectivity. A plant triggering recovery in the neuro-cognitive domain may facilitate recovery in behavioural functioning (Spaulding 1997). The therapy must be multimodal, because of the systemic nature of illness. Precisely because of connectivity, interventions in one domain are likely to encounter obstructions from other parts of the system. For instance, cognitive or behavioural patterns may quickly neutralize the plant's subtle effect.

Much of the miracle in magic – or much of the reason for disbelief in it – disappears once we take into account the self-healing capacity of living organisms and their constant search for a new equilibrium. Sukuma therapy starts from the supposition that health returns by itself after removing magical obstructions. I have discussed the daily intake of two medicinal preparations. I have shown recovery to take place within the group and within the context of a healer's cult. Later chapters will detail the initiation (within the *Chwezi* cult) and the training in magical preparations whereby patients master the sensory code behind the magical recipe. This section considers more closely the *ndagu* curse that permits the witch to corrupt the victim's protective ancestor. A later chapter will discuss the ritual removal of the curse, while in the chapter on divination we witness how a sophisticated structuring of experience gives rise to the idea of the witch.

The divination Seele performs is mediumistic. Whenever she had dreamt about a patient, she would call this person over for divination by sounding the drums. Her incantation recounted the patient's past, often in terms of unmet expectations from a kin member or ancestral spirit, and the future, often in terms of the witch's intentions. Via the oracle, she monitored the therapeutic process with the patient, adapted the medicine, decided on ritual intervention or the unlocking of chains, and could one day declare the person cured. Divination plays a pivotal role in the multimodal use of plants, behavioural measures and ritual, because it develops a transmodal stance that manages to tune into *ndagu*.

Sara is a 39-year-old mother of six children. She has never suffered from logorrhoea but she shares with Seele's patients an aetiology: the *ndagu* curse. This preoccupies the healer more than any word tagged onto the symptoms, such as *mayabu* or schizophrenia. Sara is timid and visibly weakened by her illness. Her therapeutic journey began three years ago with pain in her right thigh, which was cured with plant medicine at home. Soon after, the pain returned. It felt as if something wanted to come out of the leg. The pain ascended to chest, head and finally the whole body. Pills from the pharmacy had no result. About two years ago the pain got so bad she went for divination. Three oracles from different diviners all attributed her symptoms to a magical trap (*mitego*) that people had laid out for her and that she had stepped on. Over the years she alternated stays at two healers and two medical hospitals, but her condition only worsened. A year before we spoke she was brought to Seele for mediumistic divination. The oracle confirmed that she suffered from a *mitego* attack, which by now had fully matured. Sara was admitted at Seele's compound, where she administered a combination of hot medicine, meant to make the poison descend, and shell medicine to settle the mind. To my question about whether the latter medicine is not meant for cases of *mayabu*, a condition she did not seem to exhibit the symptoms of, Sara replied that her head had bothered her from the start. (It is my Cartesian culture that limits head-related or 'capital' disorder to mental disorder). Puss came out of wounds on her head, for which she applied plants to make it clot. Medicinal massages were done daily over the whole body. She told me her condition had improved much over the space of a year. The evidence she gave was that nowadays she could do domestic work like cooking, collecting firewood and cleaning, though to wash utensils she used only one hand. In her opinion the poison was still stuck in her chest and her left arm. Whereas this used to prevent her from sleeping, now she got a good night's rest. She thanked Seele and her assistants for having her *ndagu* curse removed twice in a ceremony that ritually expels the curse and sends it back to the witch, after placating the ancestral spirits. She said she wanted to continue with the medicine, while eagerly awaiting the day that an oracle would discharge her.

I know of no Sukuma word that is more difficult to translate than *ndagu*.[3] People say they go for divination 'to check on their *ndagu*', which would suggest the English word 'fate'. But they also refer to *ndagu* as an angry ancestor. The *ndagu* becomes visible in the chicken oracle when the protective spirit in the form of a mark on the spleen has swollen into an ulcer. A witch has sent this person an *ndagu*. Here the word carries the sense of 'spell'. It is worth noting that the English 'lots' and French *sort* in a quite similar semantic cluster mean at once spell, divination, fate, destiny and chance. I will opt for spell instead of fate because of the etymological derivation of *ndagu* from the verb *ku-lagula*, 'to treat'. So, to suffer from *ndagu* is literally to have received 'the treatment' from someone. The ominous tenor captures the idea of illness stemming from someone else's possibly justified reproach. For the illness to become that grave, one's guiding ancestral spirit must have authorized it.

The sight of the *ndagu* curse in the chicken oracle is a pivotal moment, with much cathartic potential for those present, as I frequently observed. That moment recalls the isolation commonly felt by the afflicted: the dramatic shift to a poisoned body and reproaching relatives. A medical doctor would probably hope that patients avoid the *ndagu* idiom altogether. Since Gluckman and Evans-Pritchard, ethnographers have attempted to explain to doctors that the biomedical model of bacteria and viruses does not undermine healers' epistemologies; on the contrary, its neutral language rather fails to impress for avoiding explanations (e.g. 'who sent the virus'). I argue that the demand for deeper explanations is not so much rational (as these authors claimed) but therapeutic. The hospital's biomedical classification lacks a language that could emotionally engage Sukuma patients and consider their experiential frame and the possibility of shifting away from it because biomedicine refuses to codify the world in terms that mimic the person's intense distress. The notion of *ndagu* does not evade the feasible prospect of death. *Ndagu* faces death, and therefore can set off a therapeutic process.

To decide about the right remedy, divination must determine the type of *ndagu* curse. Several types exist. Over the years I have seen the number increase and some types disappear. All are equally distressing. At the top of the list of *ndagu* spells is *ibona*, 'the piercing look'. It refers to the witch's intention of revenge: 'You think you can ignore me? You will see...' A similar type of spell is *maana*, 'the knowing': 'You will know my revenge'. *Mayabu* is commonly attributed to either of these two types. A third one is *kazoba*: the victim is 'clogged', perplexed, fearful and does not move; anything reaching the senses seems like an intrusion. The *ndwiike* curse refers to the verb *ku-idiikwa*, which means 'to be left with a burden on the head and nowhere to place it'. That is how the victim feels. A number of particularly disconcerting spells refer to the gradual wiping out of the entire household, such as *wahule*: 'They should be reduced', with a disturbingly euphemistic tenor. Diviners take a serrated liver in the chicken oracle as an indication of *wahule*. Comparable curses are *mulahi*, derived from *ku-lahila*, 'to vow', and *ndagaja*, from *ku-*

*lagajaga*, 'to topple'. An *ndagu* curse whereby someone corrupts another woman's ancestor to render her infertile is called *kajiga*, 'burner'. The witch uses a piece of cloth with the victim's menstrual blood in black magic 'burning her eggs'. *Inubo* is a southern variant on fertility obstruction, while *nyafuba* is a variant of *ibona* that is more common in Ukerewe (in the north of the Sukuma region) whose main symptom is a gradual paling of the skin until death sets in. Some Sukuma categorize *ntumbi*, the curse of someone who left a dead relative unburied for days, as an *ndagu* affliction. They admit that here no witch has intervened, but they add that what counts in *ndagu* is the anger of the ancestral spirit turning against the descendant. In this reasoning we recognize the old Bantu tradition of placating ancestral spirits in times of misfortune. (Likewise, the fertility obstructions are contemporary versions of the old *njimu* curse, which used to be attributed to maternal ancestors who had not been offered the sacrifice of a sheep.)

What do these many spells have in common? They articulate a sense of intrusion, though not just physical. Intrusion is their value, in the comprehensive visceral sense I proposed. That, we learn from the spells, is the system's state during illness. In hearing the diagnosis of *kazoba*, patients recognize their anxiety and paralysis. *Ibona* and *mana* evoke their fear of being reproached. At the same time, however, a therapeutic change is achieved. The *ndagu* spell attributes illness to the workings of someone else's magic – to something counterable with the healer's magic. The ominous attribution of *ndagu* prepares the ground for a reciprocal combat wherein the things Sukuma already have at their disposal (the healer, the clan, the village community) will be of help. Gone should be the unfathomable moral power that obsessed the individual's imagination.

The following case study clarifies the process, including group therapy, self-healing and the transmodal diagnosis defining the system as being in a state of *ndagu*. Magic recasts illness as a combat. Witchcraft discourse empowers the patient, who regains moral power after divination and after performing the right sacrifice. Consciously or not, the magic shifts code away from powerlessness and towards a more beneficial organization of modes into a system.

# Systemic, not Systematic

Albert is in his forties, a tall man of strong build, with friendly eyes, broad chin and symmetrical, sharp facial features. Every morning before sunrise one finds him clearing the paths around Seele's compound. Using a hand broom made of a bundle of grass stalks tied together by a rubber strap, he meticulously sweeps the sand paths from the entrance to the water hole a mile down the valley. He has decorated the crossroads with flags made of colourful scraps attached to poles. Flags are not a common sight in or around a healer's compound, being more appropriate to the annual dance competitions. His makeover of the compound's environment will seem awkward to neighbours and won't attract extra customers for Seele. Significantly, however, Seele did not intervene. Albert had become initiated into her medicinal tradition and as a classificatory child he has the right like any other family member to affect the environment in his way.

One morning Albert sat down with me and said he wanted to tell his story. He had prepared himself. He held a bible with a photograph sticking out, worn at the corners. In his kind low-pitched voice with a slight stutter, this is how he recounted his therapeutic journey:

> In February 1994, when living in Songila, I was sent to the healer Basole with headaches, pains in the stomach, waist and legs. Six months later I felt cured, but I was not discharged until August 1995. What had happened was that just as I was preparing to come home, my wife had fallen sick and died in childbirth. Basole advised against attending the funeral. He thought it might be a witch's trap for me to enter unprotected space. So I returned home much later. In 1997 my left foot started to hurt and swell, probably *ibaale* [translatable as bilharzia]. I consulted a healer in Nyakato. He was a Ha coming from Kigoma. His oracle revealed bewitchment by the paternal aunt. Look, here she is on the picture. It was taken at my daughter's wedding.

Albert opened his bible and removed the picture. It showed a Christian wedding party with Albert as the bride's father. The snapshot captures him behind a table full of food and drinks. He stands next to the bride receiving a present from one of the guests queing up. In the background the family sits and watches. In the middle of the first row, looking straight into the lens, sits the woman Albert pointed at.

That is my paternal aunt. The reason for her curse is jealousy over my success in marrying out my daughter in return for bridewealth. The oracle of the first healer Basole had pointed her out as well. After three months I was cured and returned home, but by 1999 I had fallen sick again. This time it was *mayabu*. I had healers coming over for treatment. Thanks to a Fipa healer from Tabora, my condition was stable. But by the end of 2003 the poison took a new form. A tooth abscess had infected my whole cheek. The swelling was big and painful. [Albert has a deep pockmark across his entire right cheek.] My uncontrolled yelling also continued a bit. So my parents brought me here. Seele's oracle showed that the problem was indeed my paternal aunt. Seele could cure the cheek. I cannot say that my head has fully calmed down yet. What worries me is that my parents have not come back to visit me. My aunt has not greeted me, ashamed as she is over her deed, which other people have confronted her with. She performed her witchcraft through a 'company' (*kampuni*) including my mother-in-law, sister-in-law and an elderly lady from my village.

Albert tells me he does not mind being photographed with his chains on. He had been able to remove the chains a few months ago, but relapsed and got into a violent row in a nearby village, so had them put on again. The week of our interview he received the good news from Seele that it was time for a definitive removal of the chains. He did not want things to go wrong this time. The clearing of paths over many months may seem like compulsive behaviour, but in Seele's eyes it prepared him for freedom and so she allowed him to do it. He had started by sweeping the entrance and progressively extended his familiarization with liberty to the water hole. He also postponed the removal of the chains until after Sunday mass, to ask his fellow believers from the village to pray for him. This Catholic minority in a village far from his home was now his only family. The removal of the chains is always a liberating event, but what he hoped for most was that his parents would visit and attend the oracle proving that the witch's threat had receded. That oracle would discharge him.

The reader may wonder. Since oracles can hardly be deemed reliable evidence, it is likely that this paternal aunt had not poisoned Albert. Not only does the diviner Seele then falsely accuse an innocent person, she also builds her treatment on nonsense. I would argue, though, that although the assumptions are not empirically verified, and thus may be incorrect (as assumptions sometimes are), they are not nonsense. They have sense, be it in expressing what the victim needs to tell but is unable to, or in pronouncing words the victim feels better from, hearing. The truth of words is less important than their effect. That too marks a systemic approach. The corollary of connecting body and mind, meaning and matter, in a system is to accept that what we convey as meaning about the system will affect that system. This is not as obvious as it sounds. If we knew that politically correct statements – such as the incommensurability of cultural values – only intensify the politically incorrect attitudes of our compatriots, would we change our statements? I doubt it. Scientists, including anthropologists, have learned to think away the effect of their words on the world. They likewise reject the diviner's words because they assume the value of diagnosis to lie in verifiable truth rather than in any presumed healing effect. However, Seele's ancestral guide often told her to perform divination outside the ritually protected compound so that the witch could overhear the oracle. The diagnosis could thus more manifestly affect the state of the system. If the witches back down after hearing their identity revealed and if the patient regains strength, then the oracle worked. If oracles are taken to be the equivalent of court cases, then diviners faking certainty about a witch's identity would be guilty of convicting an innocent person. But oracles are of another order. Clients visibly regain confidence after divination because they have sensed the guidance of the diviner and the ancestral spirit. Divination empowers patients so that they are able to greet their witch the next morning and put their trust in their protective spirit and in the possibly lethal counter-magic they respond with.

Was Albert wrong in suspecting his aunt? What counts is that the diagnosis codifies the system in a way that promises a solution. Albert had been given 'the treatment' (*ndagu*) from someone in the social network. The treatment presumably came from his father's sister, whom he pictured as envious over his wealth. For Seele's patients to believe in the treatment is treatment in itself. It shifts the mind away from the illness, as a fixed physical condition, to a social event, on which one may have impact. The therapeutic effectiveness of both magic and divination has to do with a philosophy of life that is particularly systemic. What does it mean to say that the cause of trouble is not just the illness, the poison or a virus, but the ancestor or someone in the neighbourhood or the family who performs witchcraft in response to past actions of the victim? It is to subscribe to a systemic understanding of reality. Illness and healing depend on more than bodily factors alone, for the social network is involved. Is it delusional to think so? It seems in any case that involving an extra domain of reality, one that can be impacted upon, is a useful detour to change other parts of the system that are not directly curable. Hospitals rely on biomedical categorizations that facilitate systematic treatment, just as objective evidence leads to conviction in court. Systematic means something other than systemic. The oracle is a sensorial event that keeps the client's mood systemic as it shifts attention away from fixed symptoms to what caused these and to what can be done about them. The use of plants and magic furthers the therapeutic mood. Sensory well-being can be noticed in the resolve of patients to fight their witch and take the medicine, even twice if necessary like the young man fearing a budding psychotic attack.

Following, among others, Latour (1993) and Appadurai (1996), many ethnographers have described the 'actor networks' and 'social flows' in which natural and cultural elements interact. I too trace the social lives of plants, magic and ideas in the circuits of the cultural system connecting the Great Lakes to the Swahili coast. However, Sukuma healers seem to know that change requires something entirely at odds with the paradigm of a flow, namely an intervention that freezes the system, temporarily arresting the interactive circuits – cognitive, biological, sensory – and other modes at work, to assess what they are like at that moment. Illness raises the question of what a normal versus abnormal state of the system might be. The distinction is not to be taken lightly because it faces the postmodern critique harking back to Foucault's (1975) archaeology of the clinical gaze: how to distinguish the normal from the abnormal without reverting to a value-laden, hegemonic assessment of the system? Ethnographers can hide behind the fact that they reproduce a culture's assessment; they no more than describe what Seele does when she – or at least her oracle – bypasses the postmodern critique and assesses the condition of a person as abnormal. My position however is that magic and healing ritual do not apply the binary code of normal/abnormal. Thus they epistemologically escape Foucault's critique. Healing cults conceive of bewitchment and magic as different states, and add spirit possession as yet another state. Seele herself came to regard her own illness and psychotic episodes as a 'calling', *mahugi* – a destiny announced by the ancestral spirit. A quaternary (rather than binary) sensory shift is involved that involves more than expulsion of the spell. Whereas crisis signifies an interruption of the normal course of things, the conception of illness-as-intrusion refers to a breach yet leaves open the option that this intrusion is a good thing for it shakes the victim up to reveal a world previously unknown. Initiation is the name of this structure, discussed in the next chapter.

# Not Culture-bound

Seele's patients report having experienced hallucinations, paranoid delusions as well as temporary changes of personality that point to psychotic episodes. The incapacity to fulfil cultivation or household tasks alerted clan or family members to their condition. At a later stage during treatment many patients express surprise at their previous unusual behaviour and their unawareness of this behaviour. From the frequent co-occurrence of symptoms suggesting a common pathogenesis, we may infer that we are dealing with a syndrome. Could we speak of schizophrenia? No matter how broadly categorized and possibly denuded of its medical connotations after listening to Seele, this categorization cannot be easily applied, due to culture-specific factors at play. A speech-related affliction, magically induced, strikes one as very telling of Sukuma society, where oratory is so highly valued and cultivated. A more ready temptation, therefore, may be to approach *mayabu* as an instance of what cultural psychiatry has called culture-bound syndromes. Comparison could be made with 'brain fag' syndrome, which as a variant of 'modernity stress' is specific to modern schooling pressures among West African male students.

However, the concept of culture-bound syndrome is losing its lustre (Sumathipala et al. 2004; Tseng 2006; Kirmayer and Sartorius 2007), and for good reason. It is difficult to imagine a syndrome that has no culture-specific features, precisely because of the aforementioned systemic nature of mental disorders whereby interactions between physical and social factors play an intricate role. Since schizophrenia is not a 'natural kind' (Zachar 2000), it necessarily varies between, say, Scandinavian and Mediterranean settings. Ethnocentric reasoning would be all too clear were we to assume that we were encountering a pure form of schizophrenia in our European and American hospitals as opposed to culture-bound versions in the rest of the world. Therefore this chapter followed the Sukuma classification of things, using the term schizophrenia not for a fixed set of symptoms but as a pointer to a certain state of the system. The cross-cultural significance of schizophrenia only holds at an approximate level where social, psychological and biological factors together form with an inevitable loss of specificity a structure of experience. The less specific cross-cultural categorization has the advantage of permitting exchange between therapists across cultures.

To sum up, what could we learn from Seele's approach to *mayabu*? Her success appears to follow from a systemic approach, which differs in three aspects from biomedical models. Her approach is multimodal (including biological, mental and social interventions), self-referential (diagnosis of the system changes the system itself) and transmodal: the system can be divided up into conditions (at once biological, social and mental) which it shifts between, so that certain meanings perceived in magical recipes may affect the matter of the body in a fairly predictable way. Albert's case introduces some of the main elements to be found in later chapters: gifts, witchcraft suspicions, jealousy, bridewealth, the paternal aunt, divination, and a holistic system of states. I begin by contrasting two primordial states, the coolness (*mhola*) of village initiation and the heat (*busebu*) of bewitchment, as personified in the dancer and the witch.

# Notes

1. The names of the patients are pseudonyms.
2. The few cases of *mayabu* for which no witch is revealed during divination are treated with the shell medicine only.
3. I went over several options with Pelle Brandström who spent his entire youth in the Sukuma region, but we remain doubtful to this day of an adequate translation.

# Chapter 3
# The Dancer: Gift and Sacrifice

'Aren't we all witches?' I once heard a young Sukuma man ask jokingly during a spontaneous discussion in a village bar. He knew he could rely on general consent. Most Sukuma, particularly household heads, will not deny possessing medicinal knowledge of some kind. In the evenings, by the campfire at the centre of the compound next to the cattle pen, I have often heard Lukundula and his peers making insinuations somewhat jokingly about the power of their *lukago*, their lethal magic for protection of the home. No responsible family head should be without it.

And yet, there exists another type of witch, *nogi*, whom nobody would identify with. These witches in the true sense act out of envy (*wilu*) and therefore keep their identity secret. Remarkably, it is said that these witches feel their acts are justified because their victims are 'arrogant', *badoshi*, which could be translated as 'full of themselves'. It is precisely this justified execution in name of an unspoken social law that makes the witch – almost always female, as we will see – deeply disturbing, so deeply that most deem her worthy of no better fate than death by the dismembering gashes of a machete. Public imagination, both in the West and among Sukuma, commonly portrays the witch's immorality and her transgression of taboos in nocturnal sabbaths. But what is actually despised seems to be her moralism – too much law. The general view is that transgressions are inevitable and can happen to everyone, and that there is nothing basically wrong with users of magic boasting about their power. They recall the eye-catching dancer willing to openly compete. More frightening is the witch's systematic, merciless disposition. It stands for everything a 'magical' attitude to life opposes. As this chapter illustrates, Sukuma practices of initiation, dance, greeting, alliance and magic have something in common, which they spatially express. They stimulate a dynamic, open form of social exchange avoiding precisely the perversion of law that makes negotiation and, by extension, life impossible. The next chapter will look into 'the dark side of social exchange', as Godbout (1992) succinctly defines witchcraft.

The philosophy of life emanating from the following ethnography boils down to a relation between self and world that is best captured by the Sukuma verb 'being with' (*-li na*). A Bantu language like the Sukuma language, Kisukuma, has no word for 'to have'. The meaning is composed by adding the preposition 'with' to the primary verb 'to be'. To have a wife or a house is 'to be with' a wife or a house; similarly, one 'is with thirst' or 'with anger'. This idea of having someone, something or a feeling by 'being with' them or it rather than by possessing or ingesting them is suggestive of a self tied (umbilically) to its environment without coinciding with that environment. This relational experience, whereby the self never fully owns the things (or experiences) it 'has' but is accompanied by them, surfaces in practices of marriage and alliance, status promotion and initiatory membership, which operate on the principle that there can be no gift without sacrifice. We 'are with' the world in that we give to the world and will get something in return, yet – here comes the sacrifice – without knowing what the return will be. Figures of the unknown such as spirits immanent in daily life evoke this fundamental uncertainty, this umbilical tie between self and world, the latter comprising the group. The difficulty for me as anthropologist is that Western modernity, historically rooted in an economic and urban necessity of individuals counting on their investments, has cut the tie by rendering everything calculable. Against 'being-with', it places the self at the centre as a possessor and externalizes the group as a threat – a threat to the 'truth' which individuals such as Copernicus or a Messiah carry within, for example. It recasts the unknown as the not-yet-known, an object for science. Anything else is banned to the realm of fantasy, religion or 'magic', neatly segregated from reality. Sacrifice and divination therefore do not come across to Westerners as invigorating rehabilitations of the unknown, but as evasions from reality towards the spirit realm.

Dancers magnify in a carnival-like setting the experience of 'being with', a reciprocity between self and group, whereby the group offers a stage for success and the individual depends on the group for success. The dancer's play on and inversion of social rules will in the next chapter be contrasted with the opposite: the perversion of social order into a rigid law, such as the 'tit-for-tat' calculation imputed to the witch to explain misfortune. The contrast between these perspectives on the world will grow in significance as we include other alternatives available in Sukuma society: the converting of crisis through healing ritual and oracles (Chapter 6) and the subversion of crisis in radically transformative or mystical experiences (Chapter 7).

# Dancing after the Harvest

The Sukuma calendar of cultivation and festivals follows the movement of the stars in the firmament. The first month of the calendar is October, when *ndimila* (the Pleiades) appears on the horizon. So begin the preparations of the fields. Long before dawn when children get up to herd the cattle and roam the plains, their older brothers and sisters have left the compound with empty stomachs to join their age mates of the cultivation group. Tilling the land is a disciplined activity, as much as a dance. Following the rhythm of the cantor's song, striking the tempo with the heavy iron of a worn-out hoe and the bells on his feet, the row of lined-up men and women steadily progress, only stopping when the sun gets too hot. Their body language, cries and pelvic gestures at every beat of the hoe suggest how much the act of hoeing can resemble the penetration of a pristine land being awakened from its dormant state.

A perennial source of insecurity is the rains. In colonial days the chiefs or kings (*ba-temi*) of the fifty or so chiefdoms of Sukumaland remained inside their courts during this period. Oversensitive and brooding, as it were, the king was prohibited from spilling a drop of blood lest his fecundating force, drawn from the royal ancestors, be diminished. A series of agricultural ceremonies were performed, such as the one where the queen (*ngole*) and the head counsellor (*ngabe*) would place themselves over the farmers' piles of seeds and imitate a pregnant woman in the act of birth (Millroth 1965: 171). In 1996 I witnessed near Magu the ritual shaving (*busunzula*) of the king's head. The shaving evoked the clearing of the bush. With his hair growing, the crops would too. The dehumanization of the king and his link with the land's fertility went far in the old days, I was told, so that in case of prolonged drought his counsellors were entitled to strangle him to death and have his royal tears end the drought and announce the rains.

Starting from around April, *ndimila* disappears at the horizon closely tailed by her inflamed male companion (Orion). Both finally enter their six-month honeymoon, a period in which the land casts what it has been keeping inside and fostering until then: harvest and dance (*mbina*). Then dawns a time of 'bringing together' (*kusanja*) and meeting (*kwisanga*). Everywhere, although decreasingly in the last decade, young men organize dance competitions and elders hold *wigashe* sessions, a traditional singing contest between two groups seated with their backs turned to each other. Since the beginning of the twentieth century Sukuma dancers have been enraptured by the rivalry between two secret societies, *Ba-Galu* and *Ba-Gika*, founded by two illustrious healers whose growing followings soon diffused their antagonism over the whole of Sukumaland. Except for the mediumistic society *Chweeji* (also spelled *Chwezi* or *Cwezi*) and the association of twins, all initiatory groups affiliate themselves with either (*Ba*)*Galu* or (*Ba*)*Gika*. Today, few people have been initiated into one of these societies, yet even fewer are those who do not identify themselves, for instance through their father, with one or the other (a negative third category, 'the snappers' or *ba-tinika*, is reserved for those who have affiliated with both sections). Only elders remember the specific cultural features and medicinal specializations that once divided the two societies. In practice these have become labels by which people can enact rivalry.[1] They also bear much resemblance to the way Sukuma adolescents declare allegiance to one of the two soccer teams of the country's capital, Yanga and Simba, playing over a thousand kilometres away. Even at a time when the soccer team of their own region, Mwanza, led the national league, the popularity of Yanga and Simba remained amongst Sukuma youth. The fun is in the rivalry between two recognizable fractions.

In Sukuma dance and singing competitions, the two contesting groups are of opposite affiliation: *Galu* or *Gika*. What is at stake in their battle? The attention of the public, swarming and jostling between the two sides. The group eventually attracting the largest crowd wins. More than in daily life, the objective of *mbina* is to catch the public's eye. The participants try to excite and shock the audience, and challenge and deter the opponent while pretending to dispose of the stronger medicine (*bugota*). In particular, they use recipes of 'attraction' (*samba*) said to enchant the viewers. Attraction is indeed the key to understanding what is at stake.

In the first *mbina* I witnessed in the valley near where I was living, over a thousand spectators had gathered by dusk. While one competition was still going on and the flags of both contenders fluttered, the next two groups had already begun to play the drums further down the plain. Suddenly from a grove a raging dance leader of *Galu* affiliation showed up savagely rigged out in animal skins and carrying a full-size straw doll. Swinging a machete, he challenged his opponent from the *Yeye* snake-charmers' society, of *Gika* affiliation. The crowd swarmed to the scene. They saw how the *Yeye* dancer levelled a mirror at his *Galu* opponent. The latter did not retreat. Seeing himself in the mirror he replied with the machete. He took the straw doll and slashed away at her arms, sides and head, thus evoking the ritual murder of a witch. Having noticed that he had become the centre of attention, he went on to rape the dead witch from the front and the back, following the rhythm of his drummers in the background. This scene provoked such hilarity and expectation among the spectators that they followed him en masse up to the circle of his dance group. Some of his dancers were dressed up like women and under their skirt they wore fake, oversized buttocks made of gourds. While shaking their buttocks they regaled the male spectators with inviting looks. High above the drums and audience a wooden model plane was pulled to and fro on a rope between two poles. In the meanwhile the virtuoso interplay of choreography and percussion continued. As if performing a dance of their own, parts of the audience had crossed the plain to check up on the opponent, the snake charmers' group, a hundred metres or so away. They were about to take a huge python from its case to dance with. On the margins of the show I observed an interesting scene, a dancer gesticulating as if trying to persuade another straw doll to join him in intercourse. He ran up against the reprimands of a fellow dancer, dressed up as a priest. When the priest pointed to the Bible in his hand, the young man obeyed and retreated. Then the priest snatched the doll and copulated with a triumphant sneer while holding his Bible open in one hand. In the distance I saw two men prodding their spears smeared with magic in the ground. Meanwhile, two other men were transporting a smoking barrel of local beer on their shoulders: the next contesting groups were on their way. Later in the evening, when darkness had fully settled in, the competitions came to an end and drummers kept on playing just to entertain the audience. The elders returned home leaving their spot under the big tree at the edge of the spectacle, where they had been drinking local liquor (*gongo*) since noon. Young men and women, who until then moved about in sexually segregated groups, began to mingle.

Dance and singing contests take place in open terrain. If they are not organized by a village but for commercial purposes then the groups will perform in a secluded, fenced area. The contests must take place at the outskirts of family compounds and village areas. Anyone is welcome to attend, though nobody is required to. The obscenity, open sexual advances and ostentation in the dance competitions obviously invert the diurnal normative order. They stage the urge for *bu-doshi* ('arrogance, self-centredness'), which people control and mediate in daily life and in their use of magic. This is not at all the realm of the witch as one may mistakenly assume. Against the supposition that the witch stands for the inversion of social order, like the dancer or the trickster in fables the world over, it is significant that inversion does not destroy social order, hence does not even come close to what the witch is feared to do. The dancer on the contrary illustrates how much the social order can take; how far the expression of feelings can go if performed at the right time and place. The everyday version of the dancer is *mayeeji* (from *ku-yela*, 'to walk and visit'), the 'man of the world' who expands the family's network by visiting and inviting others, gift and return-gift, and the accumulation of memberships in medicinal societies.

It is striking that in towns such as Misungwi, where outward show and self-assertion through lifestyle and wealth are common in bars, Church services and Christian weddings, the *mbina* is only a weak replica of the village's. The dances there have no vigour. Civil servants and Church members forbid the public display of obscenity. They seem to miss the villager's ease of dealing with inversion. The dance groups, who come from the villages, know that in town they should not replay the competition between the two fractions. Nor should they use magic. They put up a harmless show. This may surprise given the reputation of those places where allegedly corrupt civil servants and traders live, and farmers come on market days risking their scarce financial resources. Commercial centres are called *ng'wa nkena nguji*, 'home of the ruined buyer', or as one lakeside centre is called: 'where the home dies' (*icha kaya*). Towns are not only places of consumption, they consume. Increased urbanisation may multiply the number of neighbourhoods but the lifestyle in these is much more dependent on the national and global economy and much less mediated by seasonal cycles. The market has people talk and touch without strings attached. Such places where hierarchy is less fixed attract adolescents for the same reason as dance competitions do. And yet, if dancers would act in town festivals as they do at the outskirts of the village, applying magic and transgressing taboos, there would be outrage. Some would call them witches and possibly prosecute them. Sensitivity to the distinctions in witchcraft has eroded in town. How could one know the nuances if one has not been initiated in magic; if one actually denies village traditions the possibility of worthwhile invention? Anything deviant fits under 'the occult', denoted by the Swahili word *uchawi*. This very tendency will be seen in the literature itself on witchcraft. Written intellectual discourse belongs to a certain topos, 'a place' in the socio-experiential more than geographical sense. Modern and urban settings across the world seem to reproduce that topos. The spatial structure reveals much about the experiential structure I illustrate next. The Sukuma town has no outskirts; is an outskirts by itself, which raises the chance of nonlinear events (success, failure, crime, crisis and other instances of 'the occult') but also noises the recourse to institutional solutions (Churches, bureaucracy) and lowers the inhabitant's capacity to accept nonlinearity as a part of life (magic, traditional healing, initiatory ritual).

The dancer and the witch are alike in their use of aggressive medicine and their deviant behaviour. However, they differ in that the witch does not invert the social order but on the contrary over-emphasizes discipline, perverting the law subtending social order. The witch does not 'touch' people like a dancer but invades the body, which has inhaled, digested or trodden on her evil potion. Unlike the dancer, who suspends the rules of social distance, the witch accentuates the rules so that they are felt to be transgressed. This results in an intriguing confusion, at least in the area where I worked, between the rural (farmer's) take on witchcraft and the perspective of the Christian town-dweller.[2] The confusion is cultural and as profound as would seem likely only between people speaking different languages and living thousands of miles apart. When Christians revile the village dancers as witches, they paradoxically

73

appear to the dancers as very much witch-like themselves. My fellow villagers loved to tell outrageous rumours about the ultimate moral power (rather than traditional authority) in town: Catholic priests. They said, for instance, that their cameras could see through people's clothes, and their pictures of naked women would be exhibited in a luxury hotel in Mwanza. Furthermore, the confessional box would be the priest's place of initiation into witchcraft: certain elderly women receive absolution of their sins in return for their magical knowledge. Catholic priests somehow recall the stereotype of elderly unmarried women: they come across as a moralizing presence, denouncers of desire.[3] Whereas the priest himself may be appreciated as a person, his fixed position of superiority and moral power is not. Much of the tension would disappear were he to be domesticated in a social network of alliance through descendents, but the fact that priests are prohibited from marrying dampens hopes for such reciprocity too. If priests gave rise to a new social category, they could fit in an ominous one according to village standards.

An important, spatial feature of the distinction between dancer and witch is their respective reciprocity and fixity, and their power games and moral hierarchy. *Galu* and *Gika* groups, who informally divide Sukuma society into two social sections, compete publicly, out in the open, not covertly like the witch. This popular antagonism not only permits the participants (including the no-less active spectators) to ventilate social tensions. An interdependence is established. The overt confrontation between *Galu* and *Gika* is that of rivals who in spite of their battle know that both derive their identity from the existence of the other. They are 'relatively' opposed to each other. Each side stereotypes the other: 'The *Gika* is slow and lazy', 'The *Galu* eats like a savage and only meat'. By portraying the other as an outsider and yet entering in the same arena, they respect the other's dignity and reflexively admit that the other is an insider from the other's own perspective. Therefore, the magical combat *Galu* and *Gika* engage in has little to do with the attack and grudge of the witch. She remains a secret, absolute outsider within the group. More than just spatially, the witch will appear situated in the dark inner core of the house (the kitchen and, in the old days, the attic where food supplies were kept). We can draw up a topological schematization of moral power, which takes into account the traditional authority of the elders spending their days in the central yard of the compound (see next sections).

| Dancer: | power | relative outsider | overt competition (for attention) | outskirts |
|---|---|---|---|---|
| Witch: | moral power | absolute outsider | covert retaliation (against attention) | private |
| Elder: | authority | insider | negotiation | public |

Figure 3.1: Moral power: witch versus dancer and elder

This fairly simple scheme should suffice to undermine the literature's ready associations of witchcraft with power (as opposed to authority) and deviance (as opposed to morality). To know what witchcraft really is the opposite of, we should familiarize ourselves with the fundamentally different starting point of users of magic, which is an acceptance of contingency, also known as nonlinearity, and 'being with'. It is socially articulated in the recurring play on two opposite logics, that of gift and sacrifice. The *mbina* dance, for instance, weds these two opposite logics in the fact that no matter how much credit the triumphant dancers gain from their gifts to the audience, their new status depends on a sacrifice too, that of submitting themselves to the contingent verdict of a swarming public. Another example is greetings.

# Greetings Reproduce the Social Network

Metropolitans in Misungwi opt for the rapid Swahili greeting: *hujambo* ('how are you?') For elders and political leaders they will use the old Swahili formula of respect, *shikamoo*. These greetings resemble the lowest common denominator of 'hello' used in metropolitan spheres across the world. Sukuma greetings attempt to give each person a place in the social network (which seems to me like a genuinely cosmopolitan, rather than metropolitan attitude.) The network continuously changes with the new information obtained during the exchange of greetings. Moreover, a powerful person may rank low in terms of kinship; a senior authority suddenly becomes an equal when meeting a grandchild. Again the cultural aversion to fixed positions and absolutes comes to the fore.

In valleys with scattered compounds, two people about to cross each other's path can see each other from a distance. As they approach one another the situation is fraught with excitement and uncertainty. Greetings take care of the situation. First, people identify the time of day, pointing to a shared context, such as 'the sun has risen' (*ng'wangaluka*). Then, the junior speaker asks for the senior's clan-name, for instance *Ing'washi* (hunters' clan) or *Iminza* (royal clan). Pronouncing the clan-name acknowledges the senior's embodiment of the clan. If their extended families are allied through marriage, this is also the time to adapt the terms of address. The greeting suddenly becomes informal. This is even more so if they appear distantly related and of the same generation or two generations apart, and so stand to each other as grandparent and grandchild. Terms of address obey a dual cycle alternating between hierarchy with the parental level (address with 'father', *baba*, or 'mother', *mayu*) and equality (joking) with the grandparental generation (*guku*).

While greeting, junior men support their right hand with the left hand; junior women genuflect. The senior will ask for the name of the grandparent who founded the compound where the junior grew up, because that elder is the mediatory link with the clan and its ancestral past. He or she is the person, dead or alive, through whom the senior (male or female) speaks to the junior. If the junior is the senior party's relative, then instead of the grandparent's name the kinship term will be mentioned that defines the position this related grandparent occupies in relation to the senior party. By greeting someone 'of grandfather' (*ng'wa guku*), a condensed message is conveyed locating alter in relation to ego amidst the social network: 'You are my junior, but of the same generation, because we have the same (classificatory) grandfather'. Meanwhile, 'of father' (*ng'wa baba*) means a seniority of one generation; and the senior party says 'of me' (*ng'wa nene*) to grandchildren and their classificatory siblings.

Finally, each other's well-being is probed for: *Uli mhola? Nali mhola*, 'Are you cool?' 'I am cool'. *Mamilimo? Agene*, 'Work?' 'It's there'. *Ha kaya mhola?* 'Peace at home?' *Ulihaya kinahe? Nduhu mihayo*, 'What do you say?' 'No words', or in other words, things are fine. The probings are not fixed or devoid of content. When things are not going well, it will be mentioned. Already when slightly ill, the symptoms will be conveyed to the listener: *Nalisaata magulu*, 'My feet are hurting'; *Nigine alina swiza*, 'The child has fever'. Interlocutors are not reluctant to show their vulnerable side, even to a stranger. Instead of exchanging formalities, they are defining the situation.

They want to determine whether the state of the system is *mhola*, 'cool', meaning 'peaceful'. If the family's condition is obviously not cool, they want to point out their sufferings. It could absolve them of suspicion at the same time.

In my case, elders would ask for the name of my grandfather and say: *Ng'wa Francisi*, 'Of Francis'. Even younger interlocutors would jokingly make the attempt, so as to get me publicly to admit their seniority. Between strangers the procedure of probing their relationship can take long, as people may be family not only through marriage or adoption but through initiation in a healer's cult. We will soon come back to this informal politico-medical network of healers and cults connecting Sukuma families. The tightly knit and ever-changing nature of this network is clear as soon as one arrives at a healer's compound, where many other people besides patients can be found spending the day. One day a woman of roughly my age greeted me with the clan name of the healer. I failed to respond correctly. She remained genuflected and held my hand until my reply relieved her. To the great amusement of those around, seeing me subjected to the woman's silence, it took me several guesses and her silent rejections before I figured out to my embarrassment that I had to say: 'Of me'. She was my grandchild, for her mother had been healed by my 'sister', Seele, the healer whose brother I lived and worked with. To Sukuma those calculations on the social chessboard are very common, and taken seriously. Greetings regenerate the social network on the spot. (Still weeks after a greeting had been performed, some would discuss the correct degree of seniority after obtaining new information of distant kinship overruling age.) My friends seemed to find contentment in linking up with others and the clan's past. Likewise, they drew some form of pleasure from wearing bracelets in honour of specific ancestral spirits; maternal ancestors on the right arm, paternal ones on the left. Called 'what has preceded' (*shitongelejo*), these bracelets adorned almost any adult I knew. But they also indicated that many had at one time or another been ill and hoped such tribute to the ancestral spirit would protect them. Greetings and bracelets are a show of respect, *ikujo*, literally 'make-grow'.

In view of the following discussion, I note that the scene above weds the logics of gift and sacrifice. In the form of greeting, such as bodily posture and naming the clan, the patient's daughter acknowledged the seniority I had (via my brother Paulo). 'I was in her hands', I told Paulo; 'But you are entitled to her respect!' he retorted. She could have lost status by not reciprocating properly. Yet, in the term of address I was her grandfather; she called me *guku* and could joke with me as much as she liked. That, it seems, is the sacrifice one should be willing to make in order to enjoy the status earned. This adds a more nuanced dimension to the idea of gerontocratic rule in Africa. Sukuma elders have much authority in village councils, which decide by consensus only and have more power than the fairly aloof national, regional or district governments. Although the authority of elders is waning today, the principle remains that they depend on something unpredictable: social recognition. We enter the heart of the matter: how to get recognized by the group? The answer is the same as to how one gets magical knowledge.

## *Ihane*: Forest from within the Home

The old healer Lukundula surprised me the day he told me it was no use asking him more about his healing trade as long as I did not master the basics. I had to be initiated into the society of elders, *Bunamhala*. He was going to provide for the meat and beer, he added. For almost a year I had been doing research with healers, without actually obtaining information on the medicines and ingredients they used. All that time I had worked on the assumption that the initiation known as *ihane* had been abandoned, as it had been long ago in the southern chiefdoms. However, I soon learned that this was not the case in the chiefdoms of Bulima and Busumabu, where I worked. I have no explanation for this state of affairs, especially since these areas are much closer to the city of Mwanza. Might it be that both the district governments and the missionaries followed the same reasoning and thus never even tried to suppress magic initiation here? Other characteristics of these chiefdoms are the large discrepancy in lifestyle between commercial centres and villages. Rural areas here are marked by the absence of Swahili speakers and Muslims, the preponderance of smallholders depending on each other's assistance via association, and a higher population density attracting ritual specialists from the south seeking clientele.

I had had my share of extortion by Tanzanian bureaucrats, but it did not come close to what diviners went through. Diviners could practice their trade in Mwanza region if they pretended to do it for the purpose of 'culture', *utamaduni*, the Swahili word for folklore. The model was conservation of ethno-pharmacological knowledge. They were not supposed to be therapists using magic as their ancestors did. Not that this hindered them in any way. Those who made the effort of buying the Ward Executive Officer's 'culture permit' usually had to bribe the official, often without getting the permit anyway. Like in Cameroun and many other parts of Africa (cf. Geschiere 1997), civil servants generally have an extra reason as Christians to focus on magic as the enemy of progress. The illicitness of magic from the national perspective might explain why the actual practice of *ihane* was not a topic of public discourse. In any case, I realized that Lukundula was not reviving an old tradition for my sake as many young initiated villagers turned up to assist him. Initiating a white boy was probably an alluring prospect, but I have to say that a new world opened up for me as I was invited to more and different sorts of initiation in the area.

During a lively night, novices welcomed the society of elders with 'beer of the rib' (*walwa wa lubazu*) and everybody gathered at the house of the principal novice. I wish I could say that this wasn't me, the invisible ethnographer, but of course it was. Lukundula's family had brewed the beer (600 litres of corn-based *kindi*, and *mapuya*, a cassava and millet mixture) and his grandsons joining me were considered one generation younger. The highest rank of initiated elders (*batunda*) sat by the door, surrounded by the other *bagogo*, elders of the 'log' rank. The novices (*bahemba*), six of us, barefooted and barechested, were holding a spear or a bow. I was given Lukundula's spear. We saw over fifty members depositing their initiatory plant in a winnowing basket (*luhanga*) one by one and naming it to prove their membership. After that, nobody was allowed to stand up, and latecomers had to walk to their places squatting down. The novices sat in a line facing their elders. Then the diviner-elder organizing the ceremony stood up. He held out a rooster to perform the chicken oracle (*kuchemba ngoko*) that would verify the blessing of the ancestor over our initiation. Nobody considered this a formality. I had been warned beforehand that all our preparations could turn out to be in vain. The diviner gave the rooster to the head of the compound, who then pronounced the following eight invocations (*ku-soloja*, 'to name') in alternation with the audience's collective interjections of approval, a short, low-pitched 'huh'. I summarize the comments the diviner-elder later provided me for each invocation.

> *Bangwe, Bangwe.* [Supreme being]. I am standing east. He is on the termite hill with us, together with the big rock.

The rooster is pointed to the east, the source of knowledge and tradition, where the Balatulu (also named Tatoga or Taturu) live. The one among them who is said to have founded divination is now looking after the diviners from a height, the termite hill. Next to this invisible founding spirit stands the 'big rock', the most renowned diviner in the valley, who is present during initiation (namely Lukundula).

> *Bangwe, Bangwe.* Luhinda, of the human drum hide, to you we pray. There we went for purification.

Luhinda was a mythical ruler (and the object of much speculation in historical research), represented here as the founder of Sukuma chieftaincy. He came from the west (*ng'weli*), from an area we know as eastern Congo, Rwanda and Burundi. The west is the source of dangerous, undomesticated fertility. Luhinda's supra-human status shows from his drum, which was made of human skin. As he drummed, leaves would start to grow and the rivers would foam from the rains, so fertile a king of the land was he. In the west lie the Great Lakes. In the water, rituals are held to cleanse oracles from any sorcerous impurities. So too should our oracle be pure.

> *Bangwe, Bangwe.* And to the south we pray. He brought the jewel that we wear.

From the south come semi-precious stones and shells, which Sukuma wear as protective necklaces in accordance with tradition, to honour their forefathers.

> *Bangwe, Bangwe.* And to the Sukuma chiefdom we pray. That we may receive the power it has.

One of the fifty chiefdoms of Sukumaland is a small one called Sukuma. It lies in the north on the shore of Lake Victoria, and is said to be the first chiefdom. Hundreds of spectators had gathered in

Lukundula's courtyard, the same place where I would daily meet patients such as Albert and Alma. They all listened to these invocations of Sukuma origins.

> *Bangwe, Bangwe.* And to the Shashi we pray. That they may bring us the gourds and sell them. Let the Ikizu villager show off his powers.

The rooster is pointed to the Shashi people living in the north-east. They are venerated for introducing the craft of pottery, pots being receptacles for water. A famous rainmaker lived in the Shashi village of Ikizu.

> *Bangwe, Bangwe.* And to Kerewe we pray. That we may travel with their canoes.

The Kerewe, who live closeby, to the north on a peninsula in Lake Victoria, are said to have introduced the canoe. Sukuma are cattle-holders and farmers, but along the lake many have become fishermen.

> *Bangwe, Bangwe.* To the separated ones [ancestors] we say: as for sheltering us, shelter us then! To the separated ones we pray that they may descend. When? Today!

The elder points the rooster to the sky (*kw'igulya*). The separated ones (*ku-itama*, 'to separate above from below') are the first ancestors located in the sky. They should come down and take charge of the initiation, to protect those assembled from witches. When? The moment is now. The mood of the group is such that everybody yearns for access to that moment of ancestral support, before the initiation into magic in the forest begins.

> *Bangwe, Bangwe.* The wooden peg of the ground, that it be erect. As for cooling, when will we cool things? Today!

To cool things is to heal and to settle any lingering trouble in the village. With this final invocation, the elder directs the rooster towards the ground (*ha silili*), where a wooden peg (*lumambo*) has been inserted. I was told afterwards that the peg stands for the initiand's penis. 'Is it a metaphor (*shikolile*)?' I asked in my best Kisukuma. From my teacher's reaction I understood I had it all wrong. With the peg, or penis, our quest for magic had begun. In being erect, the peg should magically strengthen the initiand's forearm tendons (*luge*) which denote sexual potency. The forearms are said to be essential for holding the partner during intercourse. The initiated will father many children. The orientation of the rooster towards the ground is an important ending to the invocation because all medicines, as initiands soon learn, draw their healing power from what is underground, namely roots.

In these invocations the elders link the ritual not only with a supreme being and significant ancestors, but spatio-temporally with Sukuma history and with the cosmos. Eight focal points constitute the compass of the Sukuma universe, a sphere: east, west, south, north (chiefdom), north-east (Shashi), the lake (Kerewe), above (ancestors), below (roots). In each of these focal points, the unknown outside is presented as a source of power, innovation and fertility. As much as Sukuma are willing to emigrate in search of pastureland, they have a tradition of welcoming immigrants in need of a place to live, such as Haya traders from the north-west and Rwandan refugees from the west.

After these invocations, the men sat down. A murmur of expectation ran round the crowd as the diviner carefully dissected the rooster, which the principal novice had animated with his saliva. During the divination I had to squat behind the diviner and gently rub a thorn of the society's initiatory plant over his head. While I was concentrating on not wounding him, he finally gave a sigh of relief. Together with the other elders he had been looking for an internal bloodmark on the spleen of the rooster. Called *nhebe*, 'canoe seat', it signals that the ancestral spirit is present, hereby confirming ancestral support for the society's journey into the forest. One of the elders stood up, raised the chicken to the sky and declared: 'It has entered the home' (*Yajingila mu kaya*). 'When will we make things cool?' The crowd responded in unison: 'Today!'. The officiant invited each novice to sip beer from the twin gourds known as *shisabo* (also *tutolo*). The two gourds are suggestive of the fertility-through-duality played out by the *Bunamhala* society, as we will see.

So, this was going to be our moment. The novices lined up expectantly behind the teacher, each carrying a winnowing basket which we were to fill that day with all the initiatory plants. And thus we ventured into the hillocks beyond the compounds and the fields, 'into the forest' (*mu bu*) or 'to the hill' (*ku lugulu*), to appropriate the constituents of this undomesticated outside which we knew little of.

In the heat of the sun and deprived of water, we were commanded and chased by our teachers, to search for, dig and internalize the secret name and ritual meaning of some forty plants (*miji*), the details of which we vowed not to divulge. The teachers continuously 'admonished' us, which is the literal meaning of the verb *ku-hana*, from which comes *ihane*.[4] During this time we were called *ba bisebu*, literally 'of the ones who made themselves hot'. Our stay in the forest ended with each of us taking turns at crawling through an underground tunnel, which our teachers had dug. Each novice found himself in a very precarious situation while stuck in the tunnel and restrained by teachers on both sides. Then the ordeal began. (A vow of secrecy again prevents me from being more specific. I should add that those unable to stand the pain were absolved on the condition of paying a fine, as I and one other novice were relieved to find out.) Eventually the only way to survive the ordeal was for the novice to make a promise that could never be kept. The promise demanded of us by our teachers was of another order to those that were used in the homestead; it was in fact directed against the homestead. It very much reminded me and the other initiands of stories we had heard about witches and about the conditions they have to fulfil to become admitted to their sabbaths; how they order their novices to 'Go and get meat' (which refers to the killing of the father), 'Go and get vegetables' (referring to the killing of the mother), and so on. These murders would bind the candidate witch forever into evil complicity. In *ihane*, however, the novices do not keep the promise. This is the essential difference with the straightforward contract in the witch sabbath, or more generally with the devil's contract, if you will. We accepted living with a bottomless debt to the village society of elders. That is the frame of experience we created. This basic sacrifice of ours became the unspoken frame of all our further dealings with the other members of the society. I do not just mean the drinking bouts. With this frame securely in place, we could indulge in full-blown status competition. From now on any gift of beer to the society of elders would automatically correspond to personal promotion. Through these treats, young adults of the 'shrub' (*isaka*) climb up to eventually reach the rank of 'log' (*ngogo*). As elders sitting on logs, they can enjoy whatever gifts other members compete to offer. In the next section I explain how *ihane* thus joined gift and sacrifice, and established the experiential structure of magic.

After the ordeal, the other initiands and myself were anointed with a mixture of groundnuts, dug up from under the ground and burnt black. Our state was compared to that of the dead. In this state we would return to the compound and in a sense bring home the forest we came from. We returned and sneaked up on the compound, where the village had gathered, to take it by surprise. Yelling and looking belligerent, we ran through the cheering crowd and sought to plant our spears at the entrance of the house. This threshold, a 'female' space, was defended by our wives (mine included), who brandished wooden ladles. With these tools of utter receptivity, and coached by the members of the society of elderly women (*bagikulu*), our wives mercilessly chased us out of the compound. Our invasion of the home's pristine serenity, and our hasty retreat, was followed by a subdued return. Male and female parties merged in a singing procession toward the ancestral altars at the centre of the compound. Only after that fusion could we become holders of the initiatory bundle of plants that is revealingly called 'forest from within the home' (*bu ya mu kaya*).

The union of opposites refers to fertility. Thus the shape of the ceremonial beer container, the twin gourd, was explained to me in relation to the board game *isolo*, more widely known as Bao or Mancala: 'a total of one does not give birth' (*limo litabyalile*). In this strategic game the players lose their turn when their last seed lands in an empty hole where no seed lies to be picked up.[5] Life continues as long as there are pairs. The *ihane* initiation is in many ways a ritual of fertility. The rooster's entrails were mixed with the forty initiatory plants and placed in a potsherd to roast for the night. The next day the novices were incised with the concoction. After we were pulled up from the ground by our teachers, each turned with their back to us, their small fingers clenched in ours, we kicked away the cooking pot standing next to the potsherd. The other farmers rushed to collect the remainder of the *ihane* concoction. One of them told me it is fertile magic for his fields.

Later on Lukundula's brother said that the ritual itself is instrumental in calling up the rains, which indeed were much too late that year. Not that it matters for my argument, but a few days later it did start to rain heavily. Rains in this part of Tanzania are very localized. One week later an *ihane* (in which I participated this time as a teacher) in a dry area some ten kilometres away ended in a complete downpour. My friend Paulo suggested that drought has become more common as *ihane* initiations have plummeted.

The evening of our return from the forest, the diviner had taken us aside and showed us where exactly on the rooster's entrails the ancestor had approved our initiation. Each of us was given a feather. With this feather we penetrated the joint of the chicken's wing. 'This is each of you', he told us, 'on the Sukuma wing' (*inana lya kisukuma*). In principle the same initiation is held over the whole of Sukumaland. 'So', we were told, 'wherever you go, you will have fellow members who will share the food and beer of their *Bunamhala* meetings with you.' Our former selves had died in order to 'be born' (*kubyalwa*) in this medicinal society. We entered the social game. With or without initiation, people play the game. But I could imagine that by extending our sense of belonging from the kin group to the village community, the ritual did establish a change both for ourselves and for the public. From now on our deeds counted, our gifts altered the social system, our mistakes affected the socio-cosmic order. We could benefit from the power of the gift by making the sacrifice of committing ourselves to the group.

# Gift and Sacrifice

Western theories of society have no trouble recognizing the logic of the gift; namely, that some sort of society is kept in place as long as people know that for every gift sooner or later a return-gift will come. Accordingly, the Sukuma concept of *lukumo*, literally 'collection', stipulates that investment of effort and skill in the collection of social ties and goods should yield status. An entirely different concept is *lubango*, ancestral blessing. It refers to an uncontrollable factor mitigating the individual's merit of successful accumulation (but also mitigating responsibility for failure). What should challenge social theories is the experience reinforced by our initiation, of wedding this logic of sacrifice to the mentioned opposite, the logic of the gift.

Segregating sacrifice from the gift on the grounds that the former is an impure sort of logic characterizes Western modernity and capitalism which, I will argue, share a preference for gifts without sacrifice. These comprise commodity transactions that render individuals fully accountable for their actions, and life calculable (if more stressful), in contrast with the magical union of gift and sacrifice, where ancestral blessing interferes with an individual's accumulated investments and merits. The severing of this reality into a binary distinction, such as sacred and profane, or belief and fact, characterizes nation-states, both modern democracies and theocracies, all of which have an anti-magical slant, possibly because of the informal networks of magic users and the versatility of their beliefs. As a major indication of the segregation and binarism, they at the same time idealize the realm opposed to commodity transaction where sacrifice reigns in its pure state – romance, poetry, art, mystical receptivity, selfless devotion or submission (as in the word 'Islam') – in brief modernity's counterpart: sacrifices without gift. Now, to really 'get into' the meaning of magic, I argue, the main challenge is to reconnect and think together those two logics which we as moderns know in their segregated, purified state.

Western social theories suffer from purification. Adopting a mechanistic model, Searle (2006: 23) locates at the heart of society an informal contract whereby power follows once certain conditions are fulfilled. These conditions can be renegotiated, and the power can be indirect, as in a system where refraining from returning favours causes indignation and thus affects social status. Behind this informal calculus of debt and credit we recognize the social law, a universal agreement to exchange instead of steal (a wife, for instance). According to Lévi-Strauss (1949), this social law, which allows for the very possibility of society, explains the universality of the incest prohibition. For Mauss (1974), the law is exemplified by the Maori concept of *hau*, the donor's spirit within the gift. If B receives from A, then B may pass the gift on to C, who will return the favour. B unfairly enriches himself unless he attends to A. The obligation to receive and return a gift and make profit through such exchange domesticates people's capacity for violence, theft and open war. Once they have their status depend on this game, the power balance largely corresponds to the gift system.

What these theories leave out is that the system – the contract or law – could never function without something that does not belong to it: a medium. Much of the following ethnography revolves around this medium: the bride. In Sukuma society the patrilineal system's ongoing existence relies on the goodwill of the bride, who leaves her family and enters a new environment impoverished to the tune of some ten head of cattle, given by the groom's family as bridewealth. Her bridewealth will in turn allow her brothers to marry and thus her clan to participate in the gift system. She has no stake in the exchange since her children belong to her husband's clan (his bridewealth is actually calculated to pay for each child). Rather, she is the medium of, and external to, the gift system. (She is not even present during *bukombe*, the main wedding ceremony, when the cattle are handed over.) Consequently, the debt and credit of the gift system cannot domesticate her either. The reader here obtains a first inkling of her relevance in witchcraft discourse. The bride is called *ng'winga*, literally 'the leaver'. If not the logic of the gift, what logic applies to her? Her mediatory role in clan alliance and her birth-giving are like duties she fulfils. She follows the logic of what I call sacrifice.

Imagine the burden for her children or husband, had her mediation and life-giving been gifts! How could the beneficiaries ever return such an immense gift? In a sense, Sukuma culture cares for people's happiness by keeping a distinction between gift and sacrifice, thus avoiding unreasonable indebtedness. (Some may of course reply that it is unreasonable for Sukuma to subsume their women under a separate category that deprives them of a stake in the clan's social exchange.) The bottom line is that the reciprocal logic of gifts and counter-gifts tells only half the story. The main wedding song, 'Liars' (*Abalomolomo*), suggests this too: 'Cattle in return for a person! Wife-taker, do what we have always done. And that she may mature into a woman at your place.' In other words, the payment of bridewealth is a tradition. The bride obtains benefits outside the gift system, such as maturing as a woman.

The song 'Liars' warns the bride about disappointment and homesickness. It is a popular variation on an old composition in the musical tradition entitled 'The Dragging Procession' (*Selema nhutwale*). The song paints a deliberately discouraging picture of the female role in marriage (which is not uncommon in African cultures with bridewealth arrangements). The lyrics sum up all the hardships that await the bride in her new home: jealousy of other wives and in-laws, insults, hard work, false accusations of theft, intrigues, and so on. These songs are recited by the women of her family on the day before she leaves to live with her husband. She replies wisely that it is too late, the marriage has already been contracted. Now she cannot turn back nor claim that she did not know what was in store for her. I recorded the following contemporary version during the marriage of my assistant's younger brother.

The first verse describes the pain and blessing of giving birth that await the bride: the blood spilling, the bringing of water (toxaemia in

*Kubyala, mayu, kubyala.*
     *Hawiza [x2]*
     *Halina ilumbi [x2]*
*Ulushiku nalumagwa busungu, mayu,*
*naali nhaliilee. Mayu, kitabuyenze,*
*kitabuyenze, ba mayu kitabuyenze,*
*kitabuyenze. Nenhele minzi, ngwanone.*
*Mayu, kitabuyenze.*

*Ng'ombe na munhu [x2]*
*Tukaabanage sanji lelo buli.*
*Ng'ombe na munhu*

*Abalomolomo, abalomolomo!*
*Namug'atiile chumba shibili na sebule.*
*Abalomolomo!*

*Aihi, batooja mayu tubaaliile [x2]*
*Ni likili ba mayu? [x2]*
*Mayu wiizaga tung'we mabeele ha*
*nyango.*
*Ki iyiingila mayu?*
*Umayu wiizaga suki mabeele ha nyango*
*[x2]*
*Iihi babyiile mayu tubaaliile.*

*Kuja mu lugulu [x2]*
*Naanogile no ukuseenha ing'hwi*
*Kuja mu lugulu [x2]*
*Naantoje ng'wana waane buli wahabu*
*sumba [x2]*

*Ilibugumba [x2]*
*lyaaninha shoti [x2]*
*N'uku bagosha halengwa lengwagwa*
*Lyaaninha shoti n'uku bagosha*
*halengwa lengwagwa.*

*Na kale abamunhu bakakabanaga*
*ng'ombe na munhu.*
*Kakwiishaga, sanji, uyukalimisha [x2]*

*Nsanji yaane*
     *huu [x2]*
*Wa bukulu*
     *huu [x2]*
*Walubalubaga buli giiko jakugehaga*
*ng'ombe.*
*Nakongeje ja Tarime? Jingi jili*
*mabukelebe,sanji yaane.*
*Waalendelaga buli giiko waabunaagwa*
*ng'hanjo? [x2]*

To give birth, mother, to give birth,
     Is good,
     Bears gratitude.
The day I was bitten by the poison,
mother, I had not eaten,
Mother, the blood spilling [x4]
Bring me water, my dear.
Mother, the blood spilling.

Cattle and the person,
Today we should really exchange with
the intermarrier, Cattle and the person.

Liars, liars!
The family head has reserved two rooms
and a living room. Liars!

Oh, mother, cry for the parents marrying
off. What is this, mother?
Mother has come to have us share milk at
the door.
What enters, mother?
Mother has come to spill milk at the door.
Oh, the parents, mother, we should cry
for them.

Going up the hill.
I am completely exhausted collecting
firewood. Going up the hill.
Let my son get married to a young
woman.

Infertility.
It makes me run off.
And on the male side it means trouble.
It makes me run off because to men it
means trouble.

People have always exchanged cattle and
the person. Pay the price, intermarrier, so
that she [the bride] can be mature.

My intermarrier.
Yes.
Maturer.
Yes.
You have shown discontent, as if lacking
cattle.
Shall I add those of Tarime? Others stay
at Ukerewe, my intermarrier.
Why keep quiet about it?

pregnancy is also 'poison', *busungu*, in KiSukuma). The second verse confronts the ambiguity of giving cattle in return for a human. The third verse suggests that the bride's future in-laws have led her on about the husband's father providing her with the comfort of a modern house. The fourth stanza invokes the custom of peace-making between quarrelling male kin. The mother mediates by offering milk to them at the threshold of her house. Indirectly, the bride expresses how much she will miss her mother. The fifth verse voices the lamentations of an elderly lady hoping to be relieved of her chores once her son's wife has moved in. The sixth anticipates the disaster that awaits the bride if she appears to be infertile. The seventh stanza reminds both parties that paying cattle for a bride has always been the custom; the bride gains too by becoming a mature woman. The last verse evokes the uncertainties of clan alliance, and in particular the doubts of the wife-taker on whether the wife-giver is satisfied with the deal, and whether one can ever avoid the nagging feeling of being duped.

Georges Bataille (1991) was one of the few Western philosophers to have situated sacrifice outside the gift system, but he did not see how sacrifice as an external element mediated the system. He conceived of sacrifice as a wasteful outlet to channel people's desire for excess, a desire that gift circuits cannot satisfy.[6] Bataille could not imagine an experiential structure, such as the one of magic, where gift and sacrifice are interdependent, balancing the nagging sense of unsatisfied desires. Gifts have a potential for excess. A person with much capital could accumulate credit to the extent of devouring all recipients. Sacrifice curbs this destructive tendency. In *ihane* initiation, the promise of obedience to the group curbs it. In alliance, the bride's willingness to comply with tradition is an uncertain factor equally mediating male power.

With the dissolution of clan solidarity, women increasingly determine the limits as to how far the wealthy can go in giving and receiving. One anecdote may suffice to illustrate. In a neighbouring village a young woman asked to divorce soon after her marriage. Since she had not given birth yet, her husband reclaimed her bridewealth. Her mother, who had become a widow in the meantime, agreed and let the husband pick up the cattle. Not long after, however, the young woman returned to live with her husband and have children, though the mother did not attempt to retrieve the bridewealth cattle the husband had reclaimed. In response to this, the young woman's sister demanded the return of her bridewealth cattle too, and the mother quite easily gave in. So, after the death of the two sisters' father, all the bridewealth collected from their marriages disappeared to be divided among their newly established nuclear families. I was told of several such cases. Mothers and daughters put a brake on the gift system, without much pressure exerted on either side.

In retrospect it is remarkable that anthropologists since Mauss subsume sacrifice under the logic of the gift. The difference between the two cannot be underestimated. Gifts alter one's social position, ranging from subtle trade-offs affecting status, to bridewealth forging alliance, creating new relatives, in-laws, children. Sacrifice, meanwhile, changes nothing in one's social position. Honouring the ancestral spirits is a duty, for which one earns no credit. The distinction between gift (*itono*, from *ku-tona*, 'to present') and sacrifice (*shitambo*) has its respective equivalent in the distinction between *igasa*, 'debt', and *nsango*, a term referring to 'duty' (as well as 'retribution'). A father 'providing his sons with cattle to marry' (*kukwa bana*) does his duty. For this he takes no credit. Nor is he indebted to his children, or shall his kinship position change, should he lack the means to provide cattle. He will 'give them their share' (*kufunya nsango*) if he can, as his father did before him. This is sacrificial logic. Duty and share are synonymous in that consecutive generations are obliged to the clan whose wealth they share.[7] Sons should not feel indebted for the cattle they receive. 'Debt', on the other hand, is for non-kin, with whom one exchanges gifts that restructure the informal power balance (cf. Abrahams 1967: 43). Those delaying their return gift for too long will pay for it in loss of status. The creditor says to the village council about the unpaid debt: 'Let him eat it, where will it get him anyway?' (*Lekagi alye, akushika hei?*)

The distinction permeates all domains of life. A Sukuma daughter contemplating divorce will be told by her family not to worry as the bride is 'not paid for in ivory'. Cattle are, unlike her, alienable and can be returned. The contrast with ivory is marked: only the king had the right of possessing ivory, without compensation for the finder. Ivory and kingship have a sacrificial dimension in opposition to cattle and gifts. Another example of sacrificial (versus gift) logic is the sheep given by the bride's grandmother in support of her fertility. Unlike any other animal, the sheep roams the compound and can only be contained by the outer fence. It cannot be sold or exchanged, analogous with the bride's fertility to which the husband's clan obtained the mere right of usufruct. The more general rationale seems to be that when we are unable to reciprocate, as in the good fortune, talent or rain we receive, we will not feel indebted as long as we situate the givers (ancestral spirits or king) outside our gift system. There reigns duty, not debt. We relate to those entities through sacrifice instead of gift. That is the beneficial impact of sacrifice.

Of sacrifice it is said that response from the addressed ancestor can never be guaranteed. Offerings may satiate the addressed. The Sukuma word for sacrifice, *shitambo*, a hunt, evokes the hunter's risk of returning empty handed from the forest. Sacrifice indeed does not obey the social law, which prescribes reciprocity and return-gifts. The code of sacrifice instead revolves around honouring and imploring. For the ancestral spirit a token of personal attention would count much more than the value of what is sacrificed (unlike gifts made as investment). Oracles may typically request a small sacrifice of beer at the altars. In the same vein, the oracle may stipulate that the descendant wear attire (*shitongelejo*) recalling that of the ancestor in his or her lifetime.

Tacitly, of course, people expect that ceremonial dedications will commit the ancestor to protect or cure descendants. Now appears the intricate relationship of gift and sacrifice. They relate as two codes forming each other's medium. The term 'code' here refers to the explicit meaning of the practice. The term 'medium' refers to the implicit, unspoken meaning. Sacrifice has as its medium the social law, which codifies the gift. Conversely, and this renders gift and sacrifice interdependent, gifts have as their medium the sort of 'attention' that constitutes the code of sacrifice: the group's goodwill in the end decides whether one's gift counts. Unlimited accumulation may be curbed in Sukuma villages thanks to this alternation between gift and sacrifice. My explanation for the absence of unbridled capitalism is not economic or technological, in terms of what has not been invented, but cultural, hence in terms of what *is* invented, collectively, such as a cosmology or philosophy of life.

The social law of the gift system permits families to gain credit in relation to other families and thus raise their social status. The most formal version of this process is membership in initiatory societies where a certain amount of gifts of beer and meat to the group corresponds to a certain promotion. However, there is always a sacrificial or 'magical' part (which, I will argue, capitalism seeks to control or isolate), namely the consent of the group and of something else muddling up the calculus of gifts: the consent of the ancestral spirit. Indeed, on the first day of initiation we had to check the ancestor's blessing in an oracle, as well as obtaining the community's consent in a meeting of elders. Clearly, ritual initiation amounts to more than the transmission of knowledge in return for beer and fees. Each of us had to become a place for the union of opposites. Like the plant bundle we carried, we had to become a forest from within the home. The ritual illustrates the search for a balance between gift and sacrifice. It is a magical versus purifying, segregating act. Sukuma do not have mandatory initiations, but any adult man can ask to be initiated into the village society of elders. The gift/sacrifice relation is in the ordeal the novices undergo, more exactly in the promise they make, a promise they can never fulfil. After this they become 'feathers' beholden to 'the Sukuma wing', mature enough to handle magic by wedding the opposites of home and forest.

|  | Gift | Sacrifice |
| --- | --- | --- |
| Code (explicit) | Social law (debt and credit) | Recognition (contingent) |
| Medium (implicit) | Recognition | Social law |

Figure 3.2: Gift and sacrifice mediate each other

The reader may be taken aback by the philosophical turn this chapter has taken, but in my view the way to prevent an ethnography from objectifying the culture studied is by comparing and bringing out a recognizable philosophy of life. The table above schematizes the interdependence of gift and sacrifice that lies behind magic. The social law dominating the gift is the medium of sacrifice. Conversely, the recognition sought in sacrifice mediates the law of the gift. In other words, rules must be socially recognized to sanction our gifts. Magic treats the law as negotiable. I am not normally keen on using local myths to prove a point about a culture, but the cosmogony of the monster Shi'ngwengwe offers some pointers when it comes to evoking the magical attitude to life I am trying to delineate here. The myth follows the scenario of initiation. It presents the origin of the world in a transformative, cyclical (versus linear) way, for it recounts a moment of breach in a time of plenitude. Shi'ngwengwe devours all living beings, but one pregnant woman survives and her son vows to kill the monster. Despite his mother's disheartening remarks he ventures into the forest where he initiates himself into magic. There, the monster, who addresses him in a fatherly manner, challenges him to a duel. Each will have eight stones to throw at each other. The boy is named Masala Kulangwa, literally 'tricks to be taught', because of the turning point in the myth. He wins the duel because he dares to negotiate the rule imposed by the monster on who should throw the first stone. The monster gives in and throws first, but both the monster and the boy miss seven times. As the monster tries to renegotiate the throwing order for the last stone, the boy strikes his opponent. He cuts open his belly like one would slaughter a bull, and out come all the people the monster has devoured as well as the cattle which permit Sukuma to marry.

This myth, documented in the 1950s by Hendriks (1988), is not told anymore. Nowadays one can hear short parables in the village that these reproduce the relation of gift and sacrifice. For instance, in the legend of *mbago* (stump) a father who needs to travel and asks two sons to prepare his trip chooses as his heir not the elder son who domesticated the forest and cut trees to mark the shortest way (with stumps), but the younger son, who is not afraid to take detours and sleep in hospitable compounds. He is rewarded for his willingness to incur debts and for not fearing burdening his father with these debts. I have mentioned the link between the dancer and the walker, *mayeeji*, whom Sukuma men identify with. In songs, elders like to recollect their days as young cattle herders roaming the valley. As adults they put a popular proverb into practice: 'Leg is a cow, buttocks sleep without eating' (*Kugulu kuli ngombe, idako ilalija*). Only when one leaves the compound and visits other people will one have the chance of being invited for food and make deals with other villagers on the use of tools or other privileges. It takes some maturity to admit that 'the stool is in the stomach' (*isumbi lili mu nda*), namely that friendly visits can be motivated by personal gain, such as an invitation for food. The village teaches as sound what in modernity looks impure or materialistic, and what, admittedly, is becoming a new trend in marriage and business: *kumala gete*, 'to really finish', to settle accounts, which sounds more like the logic of a commodity transaction. That logic, never absent but becoming stronger now, arises from the global economy infusing the medico-political network. It conflicts with the initiated learning to accept the sacrificial side of life, to feel confident enough to contract debts, and not be too ashamed to share their problems with the extended family.[8] Next I discuss how the sacrificial shines through as well in people's attitude to their own beliefs.

# Beliefs

The verb *kubyalwa*, 'to be born', is well chosen for membership in the society of elders. Rebirth is a common theme in studies of initiation, for it can refer to new membership in the group and to terminating an unwanted condition such as illness. Rebirth can also be seen as the destabilizing of a social order in danger of becoming too static. The birth of the other initiands and myself into *Bunamhala* required an act of self-negation and absolute indebtedness. Our entry into the gift system by investing beer and meat in the group was paralleled by its opposite: our sacrifice of self, breaking with the incarcerating calculus of debt and credit. Ultimately nobody has power over anyone else. By invoking *Bangwe* or another of the many terms for 'God', Sukuma are not claiming the existence of this being. Of course I could derive a whole cosmology from the bits and pieces people told me regarding spirits, the soul or supreme beings. But that would give the wrong impression of exactitude, of beliefs defended against disbelievers. People I talked to were not interested in theological issues, and they had no authorities of religion they could refer me to. Heresy was impossible. The way they conceived of God was just one more way – next to initiation, greeting and so on – to articulate a recurring, comprehensive experience, which I have described as a relating of gift and sacrifice. Might this be an instance of the African gnosis Mudimbe (see introduction) was looking for? I dare say that it is 'magically' rather than religiously or scientifically grounded, and that this is exactly what lends it particular benefits in terms of communal solidarity. Nobody except the ancestors, silent voices, have the final say. Moreover, to return to Seele's therapy, the acceptance of uncertainty may in terms of mind-body state be beneficial as a way to reduce individual stress.

'Sukuma believe in ancestral spirits' is a deceptive statement, for it suggests creed from a book-bound religion. Discussing 'Sukuma beliefs' with Sukuma is a sobering experience. They are not used to certainties being taught (outside school or church) about things one cannot perceive or experience oneself. Such things mostly remain a matter of intuition. As a result I could never get an unequivocal and agreed-upon answer as to how a deceased person became an ancestral spirit, for instance. From the variety of answers I received I inferred that ancestorhood is probably neither an afterlife nor reincarnation in the sense of a transmigration of the soul. An acceptable hypothesis for most seemed that after death the life principle (*moyo*) disappears to be replaced by the ancestral spirit (*isamva*), which belongs to another world, invisible yet bearing on the diurnal order of descendants. Instead of a soul persisting after death, a transformation takes place by which a person becomes an ancestor. I know that rituals – whose inventions are in part intuitive – compare the living body to a pot (*nungu*) containing beer. Beer is life that comes from the ancestors, and during placation and aspersion at their altars it returns to them. After death the 'pot' breaks and becomes a potsherd (*lujo*). The relation with the guiding ancestor who protected the individual and kept them alive ends there. The traditional stool with the broad, encompassing seat represents the protective ancestor. During the funeral a stool can be split in two with an axe and thrown in the grave. At death the protective ancestor retreats from the body, which itself is left to decay to its composite state of flesh and bone. To become an ancestor one first loses one's ancestor. The deceased, as member of the world of ancestors, influences the living. As I said, the ancestors appreciate tributes to their legacy, such as descendants maintaining their traditions, habits, names and attire. There is no absolute breach between the living and the dead. Even though the body has gone, an ancestor lives on in social relations, more specifically in grandchildren, and in the fortunes and misfortunes of descendants.[9]

## Being Born

The verb *kubyalwa* is used in a second type of practice, a once-in-a-lifetime but more common than initiation: the preliminary enquiries undertaken that lead to marriage. Here too we notice a sacrificial dimension whirling its way into what might seem to be a mere matter of gift and counter-gift: cattle in return for a wife. For one thing, these enquiries have no certain outcome. When a suitor asks a man for his daughter's hand in marriage, he (and his best friend) will stay outside the woman's father's compound on his first visit. He will solemnly call out: 'We have come to be born here' (*Twizaga kubyalwa henaha*). The respectful distance precedes the 'being with' of alliance. The suitor must place himself in the passive form of 'being' born, *kubyal-wa*, the suffix signifying the passive. The daughter decides. The marriage is concluded with bridewealth, a considerable gift of some ten head of cattle to the bride's family. But there is more sacrifice accompanying this gift. The ceremonial transfer (*bukombe*) is marked by a very tense atmosphere, in which the wife-givers usually show their discontent over the deal despite the large amount of beer they were treated to the previous night. No amount of cattle can match the value of their daughter. Both parties are 'conjugators' (*bitoji*) and 'sharers' (*basanji*), although the groom's kin are seen as the main 'recipients' (*bakombe*) while the bride's kin are 'leavers' (*bawinga*). They do not hesitate to use mercantile terminology and call the marriage a deal, because they know it is not. Far from a thing sold, the bride is a *ng'winga*, a 'leaver'.[10] On leaving with their bridewealth the next day, the wife-givers will be mocked by the groom's sisters: 'Are you "men" enough to handle our cattle?'

That same mockery awaits their brother during the first nuptial night at his in-laws' place. The next morning the bride (and her friends, who listen in) make public whether he performed adequately. The bride's chaperons or 'washers' (*booja*) teased the young man the evening before by asking a high sum of *wambi*, some money to make up the bed. The bargaining of the sum is said to excite man and woman as a kind of foreplay. The public aspect of this foreplay may surprise the reader, and so may the bride's public assessment the next morning of his sexual performance. But there is a point to it: while good news provokes loud cheers among the hosts and provides the men with a meal – called 'straightening the weapon' (*bugolola shilanga*) – and after five days a fat cow ('gift to the bride-serving cultivators', *itono lya bakwilima*), the bad news will be less embarrassing than one would expect. The man is not seen as alone in this nocturnal endeavour. By this I do not refer to his wife; rather, his ancestral spirit may have let him down. (The ritual sacrifice of a goat might take care of that.) Furthermore he can count on the solidarity of the men as a group, which always remains somewhat segregated from the women's world. If sustaining the distance between the worlds of men and women sometimes feeds distrust, it also contributes to mutual excitement. Many elders, male and female, complained to me about the haste with which weddings are concluded nowadays. 'Why the increasing number of divorces?' they asked me. They went on to explain that the suitor no longer bothers to stay first at his in-laws to cultivate for them (*ku-ilima*) and to really get to know his wife and her family. This is what is meant by the husband 'being born' at his wife's place. The power of giving cattle must be combined with the duty to submit oneself to the goodwill of a foreign clan.

On the whole, Sukuma farmers do not 'have' things, kin and allies, but 'are with' these. To be initiated or marry is to 'be born' into other networks so as to extend one's own network. We have discussed some rituals and norms supporting this. Gift and sacrifice are united in the initiation ritual (promotion yet self-negation), in the wedding (bridewealth yet the bride's sacrifice) and in traditional greetings (seniority yet grandparental joking). Today the distance between male and female worlds is more easily crossed, as nuclear families form and go off to live on their own without the clans mediating. Rather than embracing a new ideology such as that of 'modernity', it could be said that Sukuma families receive less traditional and ritual support to balance gift and sacrifice.

This chapter presented dancers as epitomizing the magical balance. They sacrifice a bit of themselves in a competition without fixed outcome. They embody nonlinearity, a capricious rhythm, not a routine. Like Tanzanian hip-hop artists (see Stroeken 2005), the dancers creatively mimic, and in the same go make ironic comments about, societal trends. In the scene of the priest's rape we may read religious hypocrisy; in the preceding scene a comment about witch killings. The dancer's inversions of social order offer a morality without moralism; that is, reflexivity without the rigid quality despised in witches. The dancers put their trust in the group, whose spontaneous reactions determine the winner of the day. Although usually less manifest, it characterizes Sukuma village life as I observed it. The success of the male 'walker' (*mayeeji*) depends on those he competes with. That irremediable sort of debt is part of life.

An existential condition is suggested opposite to the neoliberal wet dream of unlimited accumulation. As the next chapters show, this balance of gift and sacrifice is, however, precarious and never fully achieved. The dancer verges on the provocative state of *ndoshi*, 'full of himself', mocking sacrifice and the need of social recognition. And there are times when women's limitation to being mediators of the gift system backfires.

# Notes

1. A parallel can be found in Ranger (1975) on Beni dance competitions opposing neighbourhoods in Swahili towns.
2. It was one of the reasons why after six months of fieldwork in a small semi-rural town I decided to move and live in a village some 15km off the road.
3. To the Aids pandemic ravaging these parts of Africa, the Catholic answer is to call for sexual restraint instead of condom use.
4. I thank Per Brandström for spelling this out to me. I am also indebted to his geographical specifications regarding the incantations. See Stroeken (2002) for information on the society of elders.
5. Better known as Bao in the rest of Tanzania, and elsewhere as Mancala, Sungka or Kalah among others, this board game is popular across Africa, the Middle East and parts of Asia. The game-play is generally described as 'sowing'. The board consists of two (or four) rows of holes, one controlled by each player. Seeds or pebbles, which no player owns as long as these circulate, move from hole to hole around the entire board. The objective is to capture most seeds. A player starts by removing all seeds from a hole and sowing these in each of the subsequent holes. If the last seed lands in an empty hole, the turn goes to the other player. Otherwise, if a strategically better hole was chosen, the player will continue sowing or capture the seeds at the last hole if they reach an agreed number.
6. Note here the resemblance with Girard's (1993) argument about human sacrifice channelling mimetic desire (see introduction).
7. The word *nsango* probably has the same stem *sanga* as the verb *ku-sanja*, 'to bring together'.
8. For those who like proverbs, here is another, which effectively silenced me after I complained to someone repeatedly asking me for monetary assistance: 'The shameful will die from a tick on his behind'.
9. More inventories of Sukuma beliefs can be found in Bösch (1930), Millroth (1965), Abrahams (1967) and Tanner (1967). The pinnacle of a legalist interpretation of culture was probably that of the sociologist Hans Cory (1953), who turned local beliefs and rules into written codes to assist

colonial administration. Culture being volatile and dynamic, by the time the book was published most of these rules transmitted and evolving in the chiefs' courts had become obsolete.

10. Bridewealth is not a woman's price but an intermediary gift to the wife-giving clan, which, as in any system of general exchange, will sooner or later obtain a woman in return from the groom's clan, if not in this generation then in one of the subsequent generations.

# Chapter 4
# Four Forms of Social Exchange

Before describing practices of magic, and interpreting them in a manner admissible to our discipline, we have one major hurdle to overcome. What if our culture's epistemology, even at its most phenomenological and non-positivistic, lacks the sensitivity to comprehend magical practices? Inhabitants of Europe, the U.S. and other places with a particular schooling system and public discursive milieu might recognize the socio-symbolic features of magical practices but miss out completely on the experiential layer, which cannot be observed and is very hard to convey. Suppose I give full reign to my Sukuma interlocutors, who describe to me a specific sensation such as peace during the use of magic; it would still raise the issue of what this sensation means for me and for other non-Sukuma readers. We could submit our descriptions of their descriptions to them, and resubmit our interpretation of their answers, and thus pride ourselves in being interpretive (Geertz 1973) and reflexive (Fabian 1983), but no tangible advance will be made as long as we do not touch on the unspoken difference that keeps our descriptions apart. The only way to avoid an infinite regress of interpretations of interpretations is to accept that the study of culture is from start to finish a comparative exercise, requiring us to consider the similarities and differences between the studied culture and the (academic) culture of those studying cultures.

Without entering into long theoretical debates I think this chapter will have enough material to suggest that the seminal sociologies of Habermas, Giddens, Luhmann and Latour rely in their analysis of modernity on a certain understanding of magic and that they have all failed to recognize the interrelation of gift and sacrifice which magic reproduces. The weak spot in studying cultures has from the onset been the possibility of radical cultural difference bedevilling our theories. I have suggested that Sukuma culture is characterized by a sacrificial dimension carefully mitigating the responsibility of the individual, whereas modernity is precisely about not mitigating, not mixing gift and sacrifice, hence about individualizing responsibility. I cannot be sure that this structure captures Sukuma experience. But on a comparative level, such as the study of 'forms of exchange', I think we can come to some consensus, namely that the modern predilection for, on the one hand, gifts without sacrifice (which render life calculable) and, on the other hand, sacrifice without gift (idealized in romantic philosophy, mystical practice and art) refers to two forms of exchange that in Sukuma culture correspond to two equally purified practices, exceptional but not absent: the construction of the witch and the practice of spirit possession. I suggest that witch construction and spirit possession, supposedly the most 'bewildering' instances of the 'occult' in Africa, fundamentally differ from Sukuma everyday magic. They fascinate Western researchers because of an alterity that is remarkably well attuned to modern purifications. The biggest challenge remains to comprehend the practice in the middle, between the two extremes: magic in the everyday, in the 'Sukuma' way.

# Modernity and Commoditization

The previous chapter demonstrated that gifts, to a neighbour, and sacrifice, to an ancestor, are two forms of social exchange, distinct yet experientially related because the code of the gift has as its medium (and implicitly requires) a sacrificial attitude: 'Will the group let my gift count?' The code of sacrifice, conversely, has gift-logic as its medium: 'Will the ancestor feel compelled by our sacrifice?'

Until now we have not spoken of commodities. How do they relate to gift and sacrifice? Critical theories traditionally oppose gift and commodity in order to discuss commoditization in modern capitalism (Gregory 1982). Ethnographers have observed that so-called traditional societies practise commodity exchange as well, if with different accents. Modernity comes in many forms. A large body of literature on globalization has underscored this plurality of 'modernities' (Gaonkar 1999; Moore and Sanders 2001; Taylor 2004), countermanding the homogenous portrayal of modernization by early critical accounts such as those by Weber, Tönnies and Heidegger, who respectively spoke about its 'iron' rationalization, *gesellschaftliche* sociality and 'denaturalizing' technology. To the latter accounts can be added those by neo-Marxists such as Marcuse and Adorno, on the capitalist economy, together with the dystopias of Orwell and Huxley which highlight the increasing alienation of individuals. These critical accounts of modernity today come across as 'nostalgic' reactions (Herzfeld 2001: 102). They remind one of ecological idealists wanting to combat the commoditization of our planet's resources and the ensuing problem of global warming by something like a return to barter. Instead of thus opposing modernity and tradition, or commodity and gift, we should speak of modernities alone and of commodities alone.

My position is neither of both. Implied in the dominant analysis is a dichotomy presuming that a critique on modernity necessarily amounts to a defence of tradition – hence the nostalgia imputed to early critiques. But what if we grant our sociological ancestors the benefit of being privileged witnesses of an unintended experiential change accompanying the socio-cultural transformation towards modernity? Their critiques struggled to articulate a contrast with the past, and were ambivalent about it. They date from the peak of modernity when a sense of contrast was still manifest and unanticipated effects of modernization could be felt. Admittedly, few of the critiques formulated a positive alternative and move forward, though Marxism was one exception. But regarding commodities, industry and technology, Marx was a modernist, not questioning the cultural values intrinsic to these means of production, whose possession the proletariat was supposed to fight over (Feenberg 1998). In other words, no theory undermined the dichotomy and linear evolution of premodern to modern. Lévi-Strauss (1962) was probably the first to react by inventing an ahistorical reality of structures where different kinds of thought could stand side by side without being hierarchically related in an evolutionary process. Yet, the price for such cognitivism was to ignore the differences that really matter to people, such as the experiential difference proper to modernity, which is informed by particular historical events. Lévi-Strauss need not have been wrong in distinguishing cognitive structures available to humans, at least if we are reflexive enough about our social construction of these structures and do not reify them into psycho-biological mechanisms innate to the human species – that is why I prefer the holistic concept of experiential frames, which are relationally defined and thus whose depth of accuracy is a matter of choice. But more significant it seems to me is the relation between these frames of experience, so that it may turn out, as I will argue, that modernity historically meant a gradual privileging of one experiential frame amongst the wider number of those available to humans.

A socially organized, if largely spontaneous effort took place, and still occurs, mobilizing an array of institutions such as schools, the media, the Church and science, all destined to limit the wider palette of experience to one type of logic. That process of purification is historical, but more generally characterizes state-led societies. It may have seemed 'artificial' in the eyes of Latour (1993), who noticed in his society, in science and technology, the desperate attempts by moderns to purify nature from culture, things from persons. This purification appears much less artificial once we realize that those impersonal categories of 'person' and 'thing' refer to an experiential segregation that moderns (including Latour) do actually maintain, that of gifts without sacrifice. One way in which social scientists could be non-modern – that is, have gift and sacrifice alternate – is by attesting to the influence of external forces (the sacrificial) on their work (their gifts). Their theories would have to build on the fact that the theories themselves (and not just the objects of study) are the product of something external to their domain. In Latour's case that would be like saying that his theory (person) is the product of a natural drive (thing). His nor any other social theory to my knowledge exhibits this level of reflexivity. Magic and art do. Anthropology could be the one discipline that keeps this radical option open. Ethnographers create a 'third position' from the exchange during fieldwork between the author's own culture and the studied culture (Strathern and Lambek 1998). This third position consists in a reflexive position that frames our theories within major cultural brackets.

Globalization studies set out to resolve the dreaded dichotomy of modernity and tradition by subsuming all cultures under one or the other category. They chose that of modernities, though they could have called them as well non-modernities, like Latour. The price for this unification is to ignore radical cultural difference. I hope to demonstrate that difference can be respected without lapsing into dichotomy. One way lies in an understanding of magical practice that does not oppose tradition to modernity, in hierarchical or evolutionary terms, but laterally relates the two on an experiential level. Thinking through gift and sacrifice, and their purified versions, will help us to make our intuitions of cultural differences explicit. This, in turn, should provide us with a comparative, instead of objectivist, ethnographic conception of magic and witchcraft.

# The Purity of Commodities and Presents

The field of globalization studies, I suggest, is predicated on the dissimulation of the experiential layer in social practice. The most effective way of undermining critiques of modernity is indeed to exclude a layer connecting modernities. An experiential layer might critically consider modernity's effect on people's well-being, for instance. In banning duality and privileging the 'many', globalization studies appear to echo the unicentric state and purification for which we invented the word 'modernity' in the first place. Because the many are variants of the one, namely modernity, the studies leave no room for fundamental epistemological opposition. Agreeing on the absence of the latter has certainly facilitated the task of social anthropologists, but to paraphrase Spivak's (1988) warning, 'diversity' in a cosmopolitan world eclipses *difference*.

To subsume traditional under modern is to obscure what 'modernities' might be the plural of, and what this singular (modernity) might be the opposite of (tradition). The unification of modern and traditional is pivotal to globalisation theory, as illustrated in a classical text by Appadurai (1986) on social exchange. In this essay, Appadurai treats the gift as a form of commodity, such that commodities form the encompassing category to which gifts belong. His proposal builds on Bourdieu's observation that both gift and commodity are motivated by self-interest. Commodities exist 'in a very wide variety of societies (though with a special intensity and salience in modern, capitalist societies)' (ibid.: 6). Given my distinction between the frames of gift and sacrifice in terms of the interdependent codes 'social law' and 'recognition', I would agree that commodity transactions belong together with gifts rather than with sacrifice. Commodity exchange and gift exchange are alike in obeying the social law. In exchange for what is given something else sooner or later comes back. Market and gift economies share this principle or code. But they differ in whether or not they acknowledge the medium implicit in gift exchange, namely social recognition. Commodity transactions do not acknowledge the role of social relationship. This we notice in two aspects of commodity exchange. First, the duration between paying the money (gift) and receiving the good (counter-gift) is short or absent. Secondly, nothing remains of the sacrificial dimension. The giver need not pay attention to the other party. (Ancestral sacrifice is an explicit form of attention.) Money and goods (or in the case of barter: two goods) slide across the counter. The exchange value of the commodity does the talking. Market officials and the judicial apparatus will endorse the money bill, backing up its credit and corresponding power. This freedom from negotiation is at odds with the indeterminacy or sacrificial side of the ritual practices we encountered.

Bargaining, where skills of ruse and seduction are played out, may be the bit of sacrifice remaining in commodity transactions at traditional markets. The virtual lack of sacrifice in commodities – their uncommon purity of privileging the social law – may explain why Sukuma markets exist at the periphery of the village, or why commodity exchange in the famous Kula ring took place in the shadow of gift exchange fostering relationships. Trobrianders told Malinowski (1922) that the return gifts from Kula partners should be made at a later date lest they resemble the mere trade of commodities. What could this mean? The counter-gift should depend not only on the partner's opening gift but also on personal aura, seduction, magical tricks, imploring. Hence, the social law codifying gifts is supplemented by its medium: a sacrificial, relational dimension containing the aspects of attention and duration, which are typically missing in a commercial transaction. So, whereas I agree with Appadurai (1986, 1996) in rejecting the dualism of gift and commodity exchange, my option would not be to unify them in one 'social flow', on a plane of many 'things' whose diverse social lives can be traced. That kind of unlimited 'diversity' cloaks certain basic experiential tensions of remarkable universality tentatively expressed by the concepts of gift, commodity and sacrifice. It is heterogeneity of a homogenous sort. The unification by a plural set, characteristic of globalization theory, denies the oppositions locally drawn. Therefore, as an alternative to unity/diversity, my option is to follow

Sukuma culture in raising the level of differentiation. To gift and commodity we shall add sacrifice and present.

From the perspective of our ethnographic material, commodity transactions seem to be gifts that lack something; namely, sacrifice. The fact that commodities share with gifts the social law could explain why the market economy almost seamlessly inserted itself in the most diverse contexts of social status production in rural communities. In market economies, however, the creditor is freed from the sacrificial dimension that makes credit contingent on the group's recognition. Hence, the hidden battle between traditional and modern economies is not on even terms. No wonder much of the social critique in Africa concerns the loss of this public control and unpredictable negotiation over social status which was entrenched in daily social exchange and which I have linked to magic as a way of life. That sacrifice – the contingency of the group's will and of the ancestor's blessing – with both its liberating and constraining impact on people, is what the market's 'invisible hand' manages to overcome, enriching the lucky few in a way suggestive of the occult (Nyamnjoh 2001). The possibility of bypassing social and ancestral blessing is also what precipitated monetization in the young generation (Nyanchama-Okemwa 2002). That nonlinear blessing is finally what postcolonial rulers have managed to circumvent through occult imagery (Mbembe 2001). If modernity comes in many varieties, those 'modernities' are clearly still the plural of something. A first step in defining this thing is to distinguish it from something else. The contrast between modern and magical 'reason' – in the broad sense of both an epistemology and a motivation in life – is this attempt.

A major obstacle to discerning the experiential distinctions and relations between gift, commodity and sacrifice is the current assumption, which Mauss (1974: 10) refrained from and warned about, that our gifts are not modernized in any way. We should realize that gifts without expectation of return are exceptional, globally speaking. They might be unique to modernities. Given the importance of reciprocity in gifts among Sukuma and other non-Western societies, it seems that 'modern' gifts (without return) should be distinguished as a fourth form of social exchange. I propose calling them 'presents'. Although they look like gifts they are in fact much closer to sacrifice. Presents could be said to characterize Western modernity, together with commodity exchange, which is their counterpart. To realize the difference between gift and present I invite the reader to imagine how awkward it would be to witness by the Christmas tree a scene common among Kula participants, to publicly complain about the value of the gift one has received, thus insisting on the other's remaining debt in relation to one's opening gift of the previous year. (I picture a cartoon in 1950s style of a man holding a pair of socks and complaining.) The giving of Christmas and anniversary presents was not practised among the Sukuma farmers and herders I lived with. Their gifts, such as beer treats, resulted in social promotion in the formal setting of the local *Bunamhala* association. Besides the pleasure of the event itself, even a simple invitation for food among friends meant an investment serving the social network. Whether or not Westerners share these motives secretly, their inclination is to consider a Sukuma farmer's disinterest in 'real' gifts as materialism; *do ut des* ('I give so that you give'). As Douglas (1994: 155) remarks in her introduction to Mauss's essay, donations (which I would categorize under sacrifice) are not gifts, not at least in Mauss's spirit of forging relations. As the moral tenor of the expression 'there is no such thing as a free lunch' suggests, Western modernities idealize the purified form and consider commoditization as the sole alternative to presents. Much cited in this respect, but never questioned for its modern argumentation, is Derrida's (1992) discussion of the gift in his essay *Given time*. It indirectly illustrates how the antithesis of commodities has impregnated the Western mind, even that of our philosophers. Derrida deconstructs gifts as impossible due to the give-and-take they belong to. He is talking of Mauss's gifts but thinking of Western presents, of pure sacrifice. The purity he expects is exactly what Sukuma gifts avoid.

In presents, 'only the thought counts'. This aspect I called attention. The intention to create debt in the recipient, as in the Kula competition of gifts, destroys the very meaning of the present. The two are lookalikes with opposite meanings. Presents are at odds with the social law's obligation to return something of more or less equal value. Most Western cultures organize Christmas presents so as to ensure the giver's anonymity and avoid all possible indebtedness: Santa Claus is the giver. (In contrast, imagine how pointless anonymity would be in the Kula exchange.) Birthday presents, with their personalized attributes telling of giver and receiver, epitomize the social-relational dimension; that is, the attention and duration that are absent in commodity transaction. Hence, just as commodities are purified forms of gift, so are presents purified forms of sacrifice. With the addition of presents a remarkably condensed interrelationship of four terms becomes evident. The relations strike one as too ethnographically embedded to retain the status of mere construct. It is the ethnographic outcome anticipated in Chapter 1 and which our theory of witchcraft cannot do without. Figure 3.2 in the previous chapter on the interdependence of gift and sacrifice (in terms of law and recognition) is specified as follows, relating four forms of social exchange.

|  | Pure gift (commodities) | Gift | Sacrifice | Pure sacrifice (presents) |
|---|---|---|---|---|
| LAW | code | code | medium | [–] |
| RELATION attention duration | [–] | medium | code | code |

Figure 4.1: Relating four frames of social exchange

At the same time, the figure illustrates the problem in our attempt as moderns to define magic. Our society privileges the two forms of exchange at the extremities of the table: commodities and presents. We are less familiar with the two forms in the middle, representing magic. Generally speaking, what modernities have in common is this severing of the interdependence between gift and sacrifice. Modernities purify social exchange into a dichotomy: commodities versus presents. The former are gifts without sacrifice (economic transaction, purified from relational value); the latter are sacrifices without gift (tokens of affection, purified from social law). Modernity's religious side, and its so-called enchantments, I subsume under the latter – crucially not under magic, unlike the literature discussed in Chapter 1.

As I could deduce from the socially desirable answers collected in a survey in 1997 for an NGO, Sukuma farmers are not unaware of the message of purification. They master the vocabulary and know when and where to use what concept. In school, 'development' (*maendeleo*, Swahili) is associated with 'self-reliance' (*kujitegemea*, Swahili). The liberation of the self is directed against clan, extended family and healing cult. Churches combat beliefs in ancestral spirits and magic.

Shops have maxims on the wall about knowing no kin. A massive, nationally organized and internationally sponsored effort during colonization and afterwards with development projects has been going on for several generations to teach Sukuma to disconnect the self from any ties that mitigate individual responsibility and render unreliable the thinker, the believer or the buyer respectively. Going by the figure above, we can speak of a disciplining of experience, since Sukuma communities seem to dispose of the wider palette of forms of exchange and accompanying frames of experience. Might Western combinatorial complexity be the product of specialization into the extreme frames? My Sukuma friends almost daily applied the experiential frame of commodity exchange, but not at the expense of making gifts and sacrifices. They also knew the experiential structure that in Western society underlies presents. A Sukuma example is the unconditional attention given by the medium to the spirit (see Chapter 8) or the 'hot' condition of novices committed to the forces of the forest during initiation (see Chapter 3). Of course, these acts of submission are not the same as Western presents. Nor are the latter equivalent to the complete submission idealized in monotheistic religions. Their similarity is structural, or relative. Their meaning derives from the intercultural comparison we make.

The figure above schematizes the cultural comparison drawn up over the last two chapters. The picture I provide is of limited resolution, because I want to keep it holistic (instead of lapsing into pluralistic juxtaposition). Within the limited resolution of this comparative picture, it can be stated that the Western dichotomy of commodity and present is a reduction of the Sukuma quaternary structure. Simply put, Western society means experiential impoverishment despite massive cultural production and 'diversity'. Globalization studies could not tell because they focus on cultural elements and their syncretism, and disregarding the experiential in culture. The middle section of the figure, relating gift and sacrifice, vanishes in societies stipulating that each domain, the public (economy) and the private (affection), should be pure in its reason. What surfaces then is a phobia of mixing. Practices that do not keep economy and affection apart are labelled in the West in terms of three categories: prostitution, corruption and materialism. Firstly, we have a hard time thinking of paid sexual intercourse that is not prostitution. The bargaining during the Sukuma nuptial night, and the erotics of the monetary in general, certainly eluded me at first. Secondly, although I would not want to downplay corruption in Tanzanian administration, Westerners may be too quick to detect impurity (and depreciate clientelism) in the friendship or presents determining the public domain of commerce and politics. Thirdly, I have often heard expatriates complain that real friendship in Africa is impossible. The social capital envisaged by gifts and attention strikes us as materialistic, even though it can hardly be unfamiliar to us.

# Sociology as Purification: Culture versus Experience

Parry and Bloch have noted that money bills are not appreciated gifts in the West, while they often are at African and Asian weddings because there the economic system 'is not a separate, amoral domain but embedded into society' (Parry and Bloch 1989: 8). Going a bit further than Cheal's (1988: 19) pair of market economy and moral economy, Parry notices the ideological impetus: 'an elaborated ideology of the "pure" gift is most likely to develop in state societies with an advanced division of labour and a significant commercial sector' (Parry 1986: 467). This idealization works in both directions: a purified give-and-take rules the social competition among moderns. That is why figure 4.1 proposes a truly cross-cultural terminology reserving the term 'pure gift' for commodities and recasting Parry's pure gift as 'pure sacrifice'.

To rephrase Parry's argument in well-known sociological terms, Western society functionally differentiated itself in subsystems such as religion, politics, economy and family, a separation of Church, State, market and the private sphere (Luhmann 1995). The assumption is that with modernity a historical transformation took place whereby a new world opened up that was inconceivable to the premodern mind. I object that macro-sociological theories disregard the experiential layer. The modern proliferation of meanings, of 'signs' in a Saussurian symbolic order, through new distinctions and further specializations did not co-occur with experiential deepening. As Frederic Jameson (1991) argues, largely in agreement with Baudrillard's (1994) concept of the simulacrum, postmodernism betrays the process the West has been stuck in since early modernity. It betrays the logic of late capitalism: a culturalist logic. It perverts

110

people's sense of the real. It leans towards emotional flatness, depthlessness, consumerism and further commoditization, and, last but not least, the decreasing possibility of any critique of this process striking a chord with the public. This accords with the purification (and hence reduction) of the experiential palette in modernization, perhaps in state formation in general. Then again, my cultural comparison with the non-modern practice of Sukuma magic noted unforeseen cross-cultural affinities, which should prompt us to disagree with the last point of Jameson's analysis. Critique of culture can strike a chord if we are willing to engage with other cultures in a way that permits them to question our own. Cultural comparison goes further than the juxtapostion in Marcus and Fischer's (1986) cultural critique.

The rituals and social institutions of the previous chapter bring out the non-discursive in experience. They reveal the relation between economy and affection. Social theories have segregated these domains. As a case in point, Habermas (1985) insists that to avoid the colonization of our life-world (communicative rationality) by the system (strategic rationality of market and State) we must keep the two rationalities apart. Habermas is modern in assuming that nothing connects the two rationalities, of commodity and present. Figure 4.1 suggests that they are respectively connected through gift and sacrifice, of which they are purifications. To come to this point sociologists would have to accept that 'non-modern' societies exist and that modern reason is a reduction of experiential frames, their own social theories attesting to the reduction.

Anthropologists sufficiently understand the ramifications of the culture concept to not mind agreeing with other social scientists that it is impossible to really get to know another culture and to enter, as it were, into the heads of other people. But there are times when the benefit of intense, longterm fieldwork becomes evident. One such instance is the study of magic. Its understanding is crucial since social scientists think of their own thought in opposition to the enchantment of the magical believer. The Sukuma user of magic represents the perennial other, much like poor Don Quixote caught in a magical world of mistaken analogies was (Foucault 2001). Therefore, sociologists of modernity, like Beck, Giddens and Lash (1994), contrast the belief in magic with the disbelief of moderns who in a tragic-heroic move have opted to live with contingency.

Sukuma would use magic as a way to retrieve a sense of certainty, and more forcefully so (as is implied by the long list of social explanations of witchcraft in the 1950s and 1990s) in disempowering times. Yet, the table of four forms of exchange shows that these social explanations exaggerate the certainty offered by magic. Magic does not adopt a transactional logic of investment and return. I have sufficiently pointed instead to the alternation of gift and sacrifice in magic. Illustrative of transactional logic are technologies such as hoes or radios, and these Sukuma farmers have too. Quite contrary to the sociological view, the principle of magic is not such certainty. It is contingency – the unsure 'arrival' of events. Contingency (from the Latin *contingere*, 'to arrive') prevails not only in the magical recipe's symbolic additives, but also in the experiential condition stimulated in the user. If anything distinguishes *ihane* initiates from moderns, it is that the former live contingency, rather than struggling with it like a companion they are uncomfortable with.

The concepts heading Figure 4.1 – commodity, gift, sacrifice, and present – are cultural labels for practices that differ much within and across communities. Other terms may have been better. What is universal are the relations between the terms. The experiential connections (proposed in terms of code and medium) underneath the four headings make up the table. When we describe the flow – Appadurai's social flow of things – by which a thing such as beer transforms, depending on the context, from a present to a commodity, and then again to a gift or a sacrifice, we are talking of shifts between fixed categories. True, the categories are relative; they could be replaced by a wider range of more specific categories. But within a given depth of comparison, such as the fourfold one in our table, the relations between the labels heading the table are fixed. They have the advantage over a list of various 'modernities' that they speak the same language. They are mutually exclusive and exhaust all possibilities, and this in a less shallow manner than the binary distinction of modern/tradional (non-modern). Accordingly, we no longer need to oppose witchcraft to modernity. Nor should we revert to the contrary, as in contemporary studies discussed in the introduction, either likening modernity to magic or approaching different magicalities as forms of modernity. To take forms of social exchange as a starting point permits us to extend the analysis to all societies. Each form connects economic relations to cultural (including religious) beliefs, which results in a set of four potential 'moral economies'.

The hermeneutic circle sums up the phenomenological take on culture I have adhered to. The meaning of a part exists in its relation to the whole (Gadamer 2004). In this study the whole is *anthropos*, rather than 'a' culture or one modernity independent of others. The picture of social exchange offered in Figure 4.1 is low in resolution, but it pictures the whole and its parts, so that Sukuma culture and my own can be compared. The four combinations of code and medium are part–whole relations that distinguish and connect four socially grounded frames (structures) that will help us in characterizing four categories of so-called religious practice central to our ethnography: magic and initiation, witch construction, divination and healing, and finally spirit possession. The frames of experience proposed by Goffman (1974: 13) and Bateson (1990: 187) were products of the phenomenological tradition. They described how frames such as 'work', 'interview' or 'play' organize people's experience and communication. However, their specificity qua social domain concealed interrelations. A quaternary structure of forms of exchange seems shallow, but it is an advance in relation to the dual structure of former comparative analyses.

One type of comparative analysis I have mentioned is cultural critique such as Marcus and Fischer's (1986). My comparison grounds critique as well, but it does not do so by juxtaposing the author's Western culture to 'the' Sukuma culture, opposing gift to commodity societies. I have illustrated the riposte by globalization studies to the naivety of cultural critique. They return to a unitary structure of heterogeneity excluding opposite frames. The move is advantageous for a globalist analysis, but hampers the understanding of cultures. The fourfold differentiation of Figure 4.1 proceeds in the other direction. To do our job as ethnographers we should not hide ourselves behind descriptive data, as if cultures and their members speak for themselves. A culture cannot be added to 'the ethnographic record' without considering the relationship between cultures. It is important to note that any such relationship requires an a-historical dimension in the analysis and thus will remain largely elided as long as our analysis sticks to the ethnographic present (cf. Fabian 1983) and fears to approach anything cultural as out of time. Fabian's critique of anthropology did not point to novel ways of analysis and thus had an impoverishing effect for diminishing our capacity to compare and differentiate cultures, which used to distinguish anthropologists from sociologists and led them to travel and seek epistemological challenges. To not map the topoi or structures underlying our descriptions has been counterproductive because the intention was to become reflexive about our analysis. Furthermore, the focus on the ethnographic 'here and now' as the one connection between self and other has resulted in a generalized sense of difference. Any suggestion of an inherent affinity between European positivism and Sukuma witch-construction (through the concept of moral power) will seem controversial. There would be no way for a Sukuma and me to meet for real unless through speech acts negotiating our differences in the now (or through a biogenetic universal). Not unlike quantitative sociologists presuming surveys to convey meaning, we thus treat culture as the sum of opinions expressed by individuals. Instead, this book proposes the hard and always incomplete work of cultural comparison, whereby meanings are observed practices cast and related in terms of the author's culture. Without an eye for this a-historical dimension, for these unconscious patterns of relating, we pretend to be objective describers without cultures of our own.

Fieldworkers do this work by immersing themselves in a new cultural perspective. The ethnographer observes practices (see p in Figure 4.2, below) and after participating and comparing them eventually accords experiences (see e, below) to these practices. I am not claiming we plumb the depths of a subject's concrete experience. It is, more modestly, the relative and structural reality of frames of experience we are talking about. These structures reveal that apparently similar cultural practices, such as magic and witch construction, can be radically different in experience and, conversely, that distinct practices such as witch construction and scientific explanations can be similar in experience. By experience I mean more generally the frame predicting a person's action. For instance, during the first three months of my fieldwork, I spent most of my time in a small town with the personnel of an NGO I had initially collaborated with. On our informal evenings I first heard about the problem of witchcraft. Some educated Tanzanian colleagues assumed that in distant villages with little government control or Western influence, witch killings were rampant. When I later moved to live in a village and heard my neighbours talk of a certain woman as a witch, I feared the worst. Schematically put, I registered people's practice of saying 'she is a witch' (p1, below). An oracle had evidently confirmed my neighbour's suspicion of witchcraft. A year went by, but the woman in question was not killed. By that time I had observed many such instances of suspicion and divination without these leading to violence. I became aware of my own culture, of the experiential frame (e1) that accompanied the words 'she is a witch' (p1) for me and for the NGO workers. We interpreted those words within the fairly Western frame of absolute truth, which law courts and science strive for. Within this frame, p1 amounted to witch killing. An irremediably evil person was identified. Why did Sukuma in the village not kill her? Because their frame was different, I learned. The statement 'she is a witch' (p1) was combined with the experiential frame of magic: 'We are all users of magic, and I have strong protection' (e2). The result was not execution of the witch, as predicted from my experience (e1).

$$m = \frac{p_1 + p_2 + p_3 + \dots}{e_1 + e_2 + e_3 + \dots}$$

Figure 4.2: Meaning as the holistic relation of practice and experience

In brief, similar statements on witchcraft (p1) appear to have different meanings (m) once we include experiences (e1 and e2). The two ellipses in the formula illustrate this. Ellipse p1/e1 stands for the meaning of witchcraft in a positivist frame, while ellipse p1/e2 stands for the very different meaning of witchcraft in a magical frame. I contend that the problem of witchcraft studies has been their inclination to the first frame. Meaning, the unit of our cultural analyses according to Geertz (1973), consists of both practice (p) and experience (e). Sociologists of a praxiological slant such as Bourdieu stick to practice.

The rapport between practice and experience generates culture. Now, the temptation may be to mechanistically reconstruct culture: combine p1 and e2 and we would obtain the Sukuma meaning of witchcraft. As the formula above illustrates through the ellipsis punctuation mark designating infinity (above and below the fraction bar), this will not do because meaning (m) only exists as a relation. It cannot be disconnected from all other practices and experiences in the formula. Therefore, we have to limit the terms in our equation. Unfortunately we have to limit the resolution to keep the picture holistic. Not one definition I might have given – of witchcraft, the gift, and so on – could be absolute. While my ethnographic data seek to reconstruct a practice from bits and details to their general meaning, my interpretation proceeds in the other direction, dividing up the whole of social exchange into structures.

Of equal importance to differentiating what looks the same is discovering similarity between distinct practices. Chapter 7 will suggest that witch killings and science bear an unexpected resemblance. While the disciplining of experiential frames towards a calculable type may have propelled technological discovery in Europe, it must have had grave consequences in other domains. The practice of identifying evil (p1) became endowed with the aura of truth (e1). This certainty allowed for the systematic execution of suspects. In the magical frame (e2) prior to the witch-craze it apparently did less. Many innocent people were burned at the stake at the birth of the experiential disciplining known as modernity. It took a traumatizing witch-craze before the practice of naming witches stopped. Modern disciplining framed witchcraft beliefs into a meaning (p1/e1) that was socially unsustainable. It may explain the rapid dissimulation of these beliefs in Europe after a violent transition period when experience had changed while practice had not (that is, until the frame of truth, e1, found the scientific procedures to match, which would be p2).

I will show later on that this analysis, distinguishing practices and experiental frames, confronts anthropologists who associate Sukuma farmers with witch killings and propose more education and development as a solution. My data predict negative consequences of such stimulation of the positivist frame, as long as the practices and beliefs have not changed by themselves. What was once a magical experience becomes an instance of truth to act on.[1] Unfortunately, this analysis has become harder to substantiate as the concept of culture goes out of fashion and cultural difference loses its experiential depth in favour of global diversity. Anyone said to fundamentally differ, as in bearing a magical attitude to life, is thought to be excluded from the only frame that counts for humanity. That is when sociological analysis begins to suffer from modernity's disciplining of experience, from its contraction of thought to a unitary frame.

By disregarding experiential oppositions, a unitary frame prevails, not surprisingly a once-unwanted guest: self-interest (desire or power) becomes the fundamental human motive. Although Bourdieu (1979) did not intend it, in his 'social distinction' the worldly wise motive of self-interest cements the whole edifice of social classes and trajectories. Postcolonial literature has also been replete with this motive, cast in terms of power/resistance. Thus the social sciences have been instrumental in modernity's purification. People making choices based on intuition or a sense of destiny would be negligible exceptions. They would belong to a separate category containing religiosity, superstition and magical beliefs. Again we find ourselves at the two extremes of Figure 4.1, with the emphasis on the lefthand column. Power logic, an antagonistic experience in which '[a]ctions ... produce their opposites', dominates the anthropological interpretation of culture in the era of globalization, as attested to by various definitions: the 'assertion of cultural distinctiveness', the 'indigenization of modernity', 'the localizing of the global' (Sahlins 1999: 410).[2] Appadurai (1996) conceives of rituals as 'producing locality'. Rituals such as funerals are meant to assert the group within the global world (what happened to coping with bereavement?). Again we encounter power, one type of micro-relation that is inflated to a macro-social analysis of global processes.

My proposal has not been to offer a unitary structure alternative to 'power', but to deepen the structure after considering another epistemology. The idea of 'being with', which *ihane* initiation and other instances of the magical structure prepared us for, incorporates opposite meanings, such as the capacity to contract debts, to concoct magic, to compete, and to overcome the fear of arousing envy. One structure relates to all the other structures, as in Figure 4.1. When my Sukuma neighbour told me about the problem of conceitedness (*bu-doshi*) arousing the witch's wrath, I asked him who would tell him if he was becoming *n-doshi*. He smiled at me: 'Nobody will tell you. You will just go on living together' (*Batukuluubila. Kwa hiyo ukubi nabo shihamo duhu*). Thinking of the functionalist theory of witchcraft as a levelling force (and as an obstacle to development), I said to him jokingly that he had better watch out about wearing fancy clothes. To my transactional logic he laconically replied with an attitude wedding gift and sacrifice : 'Oh, to wear them, I will wear them all right. But while fearing!' (*Yuu, kuzwala, nakuzwaala. Aliyo nakoogoha!*). His magical frame of 'being with' was not a faint, sort of animistic perspective on the world. It incorporated the possibility of witchcraft and levelling, the main thrust of functionalist theory, and went beyond it. My neighbour was telling me that backing out in the face of an imaginary envious community is not a cool attitude; is not worthy of a bearer of the 'forest from within the home'. The next chapter examines this problematic, 'hot' experience, when moral power originates.

# Notes

1.  I will briefly discuss the witch-hunts in Europe, as well as the genocide to the west of the Sukuma region in the much more educated and Christianized region of Rwanda and Burundi; see Chapter 7.
2.  Here Sahlins is respectively citing and agreeing with Strathern, Hannerz and Appadurai.

# Chapter 5
# The Witch: Moral Power and Intrusion

Before leaving for my fieldwork in Tanzania, I adhered to the uncontroversial view of the witch being in essence a deviant, marginal figure, an outsider isolated by an accusing community. Therefore I was somewhat apprehensive about my future position in the community. What if misfortune or accident were at some time imputed to my presence? In the village I quickly came to realize that it was exactly that I did not belong, my exteriority, which reassured the community. 'The witch resides within the home' (*Nogi ali mu kaya*), I heard Paulo say. It is not just that the wealth white people are assumed to have helps against suspicions of jealousy. An outsider who has little in common will not be expected to feel any jealousy or have a motive. Strangers do not bewitch, they enchant.

The word for stranger is *misa*, 'the hidden' (from *ku-bisa*, to hide). Bewitchment requires a great deal of secrecy. The hidden evokes the occult, a concept that does not cease to thrill postcolonial anthropologists. However, for 'the hidden' to evoke lethal witchcraft, it must be wedded to its opposite, 'wombness' (*buda*), which is a Sukuma synonym for kinship (*budugu*). The reasoning is that the descendant does not die without the consent of the ancestor. The ancestor embodies, so to speak, the wish of the anonymous collective – the 'people' or the 'group'. Witch and angry ancestor were often mentioned together in Lukundula's compound. The witch supposedly says about her victims: 'I won't give them back. The python does not throw up what it has swallowed!' (*Natubinhaga. Isato ulu yumila itaswaga!*) The metaphor of the python as inverted womb captures the dark side of kinship. Motherhood can be a moral basis for power over other persons. The following pages discuss this intrusive quality of bewitchment. The

119

meaning of words depends on experiential frames. I will try to reconstruct these through fragments of recorded conversations.

The witch is an absolute outsider within – kin (or allied) yet an absolute other in her evil motive and in the secrecy of her action (therefore, she is an Other). As a member of the same social and normative system, the witch is entitled to compare. While an insider, she is an opponent. This sums up the feeling of intrusion proper to bewitchment. To be able to kill, the witch must partake of the system, the scheme set up by the founding fathers of society. My friends in the village did not use the standard term *nogi* to speak of a witch, unless jokingly. Instead they used the more sophisticated *ng'wiboneeji*, generally meaning an 'evildoer' (like its Swahili counterpart *mwoneaji*), but expressing a more complex sentiment going by the grammatical structure built around the stem *-bon*, 'looking', and more exactly *-ibon*, 'seeing oneself'. The grammatical structure reflects the structure of experience, which, to anticipate our later discussion, has several aspects, such as looking down on someone, an envious look after comparison, and a warning from the envious about what the envied will get to see.

In this vein Tanzania's villagization policy of the 1970s should be reconsidered. People told me that spatial centralization into monocentric communities inadvertently boosted the list of suspects as well as the motives for witchcraft. Neighbours who formerly enchanted outsiders and lived apart from them at a distance conducive to social exchange, alliance and greeting (see Chapter 3) now became almost as socially relevant as family members. Consequently, neighbours were increasingly considered to be emotionally involved with and to belong to the group of insiders.

# Measures of Protection

The dancer and the witch stand for two realities of witchcraft. The first stems from the perspective of members of society caught up in the community's ongoing informal game of power and status acquisition, in which expansive social networks and updated medicinal knowledge help. Men and women, especially professional healers, possess magic to fight off rivals and win over newcomers in the village. Good and evil are a matter of who is winning. The other perspective is that of members of society – the same members just mentioned but on other occasions – who suffer an episode of powerlessness. They will consult diviners and thus wind up at the places where I worked, healers' compounds. Those completely deprived of the means to further participate in society become patients in search of new magic.

Healers (*bafumu*) swiftly shift between both registers of witchcraft. For the dancer's frame of experience, let us attend to the words of a male healer in his early fifties:

> The problems I have had since I started giving therapy are many. At night an owl came to land on my house and it died on the spot. Then one night a jackal came. When it arrived at the entrance of the compound it just died there. It did not even reach the central yard. When I woke up in the morning I found the corpse. Sometimes birds die as soon as they land on my yard. One time my cattle had escaped from the pen. All of them had gone astray at night. I looked for them in vain, until noon when I caught up with them far away. Furthermore, hyenas came, two of them. When they approached my compound, they stopped at the edge. They turned back without doing anything and went to the pond to wash themselves. And many nights I have dreamt that an elderly woman called me outside. But when I came out, there was nobody. When going back to sleep, you dream again, then go outside and fail to see anything. But you know that person. Yet, when you come out, she is gone. Those are the problems I have had to deal with as a therapist.

This healer is telling us that his compound has regularly been under attack, attacks of an occult nature. They occurred at night and in the form of scavenging, nocturnal, wild animals, such as the owl, jackal and hyena. These are not just any owls or hyenas but accomplices sent by the witch. Birds too can be used as carriers of lethal sorcery. While ventilating his frustration over these attacks, the healer asserts the power of his protective medicine, *lukago* (from *ku-kaga*, to protect). He is actually boasting about the number of intruders that have succumbed to his defences. His place is a safe one for patients. Defensive yet lethal, the *lukago* remedy consists of small, black rock-like sediments of roasted ingredients of plants and animals that are associated with death. Some claim that one of its ingredients should be a part, no matter how small, of the sexual organ of an executed witch. (Nobody considered this an essential *shingila*, 'access'; it may be a new invention to counter the increasingly strong attacks of contemporary witches.) The *lukago* remedy is used preventively for the protection of body and compound through insertions in the ground around and within the homestead, in its thresholds, open fire and hearth, followed by strategic incisions to insert the same concoction on the fontanel, chest, armpits, belly and feet of the household members. Anyone trespassing with evil intentions or carrying aggressive magic should succumb on the spot. The reasoning is that one cannot be blamed for magically warding off and possibly killing an intruder.

There also exist non-lethal types of magical protection. Some of the potions one can buy from a healer are *lihumuja* (to prevent quarrels at home), *isalang'hanya* (to make intruders quarrel), *shitahewa* (to prevent failure of medicine), *bulemela* (to disarm an opponent), *ilegi* (to chase ill-intended visitors away with neck lumps; a remedy adopted from Haya people in Bukoba area) and *majimijo* (from *ku-jimija*, 'to lose': in its proximity all evil magic in a homestead loses its power). Healers make from these; many are in the business of selling new protective concoctions or recipes, which they claim to have updated in reaction to of the latest innovations of witches. From this perspective there is no fundamental difference between healers and witches. They operate in the same arena and are thought to probably learn from each other. Clients expect this from their healers in their increasingly globalized world, connected to innovations in remote places. In the village where I lived one elderly woman accused of bewitchment was said to stay over at the healer's compound to share some of her knowledge in return.

The healer quoted above talked of intrusions into his compound. Yet, in neither of his examples did the threat originate from within. It proceeded from the outside towards the inside, into the home. None of the attacks proved fatal to him. The intruders died. Their power dissolved the moment they reached the limits of the compound, either its entrance, roofs or ground. Even the hyenas, who like jackals and certain birds can act as a witch's messengers, noticed these limits and fled to wash away the *lukago* they had encountered there. In the healer's dream the elderly lady remained outside. He knew her. She was an identifiable opponent challenging him. She was haunting him, yet without the personal, intrusive quality recounted by Seele's *mayabu* patients.

# The Absolute Outsider Within

Unlike Evans-Pritchard's (1976: 226ff) famous Zande witch, whose deadly force is activated unconsciously, the Sukuma witch carries out her secret projects deliberately and in collaboration with others. Her outsidership is absolute in that her actions are hidden and non-reciprocal. No one can exchange with the witch, unless one gives up one's social identity to become a witch, zombie or professional healer (*mfumu*) with the obligation of getting to know the witch's potions and finding their antidotes.

There are at least five types of attack, all of which accomplish a form of intrusion, unnoticeably bringing in a harmful substance. The most common two are inserting a magical potion in food (*ku-lisha*, to feed) and placing a snare (*ntego*, plural: *mitego*) on the road (*ku-pandya*, to cause to step on). Three more methods of intrusion are to travel invisibly and reach the victim via natural phenomena such as whirlwinds (*shululu*; cf. the so-called *huluhumbi* curse), to verbally transmit the curse by secretly pointing (*ku-sonela*) at the victim (a recent variant is the well-known act of blowing over one's hand), and throwing (*kuponya*) the harmful substance from a distance. The latter type is subdivided into 'throwing a little murder' (*kuponya (tu)lubugu*), 'throwing an earthen ball' (*kuponya sululu*) and 'throwing sticks' (*kuponya shiti*). In the first the witch smears a black concoction on four twigs of the *mbudeka* tree (from *ku-budeka*, to break) and throws these in the four directions of the compass, with the last stick broken as a metonymic act of killing. In the second a black concoction is inserted in a small earthen ball, to be flung with a flexible stick from a distance into the victim's homestead. (Sukuma from the eastern Ntuzu region call this *nhabigi*.) The third is a medicinally anointed piece of wood hidden in the belongings of emigrants, making them the focal point of the witches in their new neighbourhood.

The family's protective medicine (*lukago*) may turn out to be no match for this sophisticated technology of warfare and communication. Healers try to keep up and 'dream' accurately, their medicines adopting the same main principle as the witches'. They mix plants with *shingila*, metonymic representations of the subject (the patient in the case of healing, the victim in the case of witchcraft). Healers and witches are alike in hunting with invisible traps. Healers also live at the periphery of the village. It has tempted many a study to liken them. However, the witch fundamentally differs from the healer in the quality of insidership she combines with outsidership. Not only is she an absolute outsider one cannot exchange with, she operates from within the intimacy of the family or the homestead. The witch has to 'know' (*ku-mana*) the victim, in the sense of having access. The ingredient of 'access', *shingila*, is therefore essential (see Chapter 9). One kind of access is kinship, 'wombness'. The authority of kin is amplified if combined with seniority. A second kind of access emanates from the gift system, when it falters and leaves someone with an irremediable debt. The Sukuma word for credit, *shili*, refers to something that 'feeds', possibly referring to the condition of the indebted as being eaten. Reproach following the violation of shared norms such as solidarity and hospitality may also provide the entitlement and thus the access a witch needs to kill. The moral dimension endows the untamed exteriority of her recipes with an intimacy corrupting the ancestral spirits and the house's protective magic. The absolute outside furnishes power; the absolute inside furnishes morality. Together they constitute the moral power the witch draws on. The healing rituals, magic and divination that we will discuss serve to harness and redirect moral power. It is a type of power beyond domestication. Chapter 7 will ask if that might be why Western society erased its name.

# A Sensory Reality

The intrusion of witchcraft is first and foremost a sensory experience. The intrusion can be aural – nocturnal sounds, whispers, pebbles brushing the roof at night, or the laugh of a hyena can indicate attacks. It can also be visual, seen by the victim on the faces of the witch's accomplices silently staring. It is worth noting here that the most common attack is *ibona*, a 'vengeful look' ('seeing', *-bona*, forms the word stem). The witch has pointed to ego while whispering: 'You will see my revenge'. The reciprocal and receptive vision, which seeks contact with outsiders in a greeting or an invitation to watch one's dance, has been replaced by an invasive seeing in probably the most active form imaginable, a reproachful, silent stare that kills. *Bonekagi*, the cook says, 'Have a look', when serving the evening meal on a big plate for the men to share. This subtle everyday play on attraction and distance, described in Chapter 3 in practices of 'being with', has been perverted by witchcraft into a poisonous invasion of permeable bodies.

Starting from this sensory frame, the diviner carefully opens up a bird to check for defects such as bruises, ulcers and tears (see Chapter 7). The entrails show whether poison has entered the body. Did it enter through the mouth, the diviner asks, or the feet? The snares and potions break the rule of distance. Part and parcel of that sensory reality is the moral access the diviner detects. The most common way of talking about this moral power is in terms of envy and people's anger over someone's *budoshi*, 'conceitedness'. In the next section I will tease apart this second perspective on the witch via fragments of private conversations I recorded (with my informants' permission). Interviewers create by their presence a public setting, which calls for impersonal and often fantastic stories. One such tale in Tanzania concerns the ghost village of Gamboshi, where Sukuma witches hold their sabbaths (Stroeken 2001). The stories are not what preoccupy real people in real situations. Only in the privacy of the respondent's room, and after long-term participation in the community, did the stories begin to differ substantially in tenor and bring home the patient's perspective.

## *Budoshi*: Arousing Jealousy

To illustrate the second register of discourse and experience, that of 'the witch' proper, consider the following episode from a young teacher's life. He narrated it to me many years later, one afternoon in the company of friends. After having spent his entire youth in the village, he had studied in town to become a teacher, an experience which changed him as a person. But the return was a bigger shock. He had been assigned to a teaching post in a primary school, some fifty miles away from his native village. While there he began to feel more and more uncomfortable in the relative isolation proper to a schoolteacher's life in the village. Schools are built on a community's periphery, with a curriculum not exactly adapted to the Sukuma cultivator's preoccupations. One day a healer passed by to caution him about the prevailing dangers. The healer gave the teacher *wija* medicine to perceive the invisible and alert him in case witches were near. With a medicinal concoction he would be able to chase them away. So intense had his anxiety become in the meantime – villagers' conversations had in his eyes taken the shape of relentless backbiting directed at him – that, triggered by severe drunkenness and the healer's warning, one night he saw his neighbours gathering in and around his homestead like witches performing their sabbath, with a niece of his entering his sleeping room. The next day, he recounted, he packed his bags, left the school and requested a transfer.

Underlying the teacher's mind-boggling portrait of the transgressive behaviour of others, we find that the witches are not outsiders or marginal figures. They are everyday people representing the group itself. This witchcraft fantasy is not uncommon. It plays on an intricate shift of perspective and perhaps on the very idea of cultural difference. In the fantasy we recognize the individual imagining being sanctioned by the group, since the invaders seem evil only to him while they represent the group and its dominant morality from which the individual deviates. At this point of the analysis it is crucial not to fall into the trap found in functionalist studies of the 1950s of considering the community as an acting body with seething levelling pressures, persecuting individuals that stand out. The teacher feels the structurally intrusive position he is in with regard to the community, or – from his point of view – the community is in regarding him. His fear of intrusion and social exclusion does not agree well with the community's everyday polycentric complex of social exchange I portrayed earlier. Suspecting others of envying you to the point of murder does not befit the polycentric complex, where personal freedom and varying levels of success are permitted and even expected from everyone. To seriously label someone else as too successful or self-important is in itself a suspicious act. Still, the teacher feared he had given cause for such a reproach among his fellow villagers.

Here we can begin to see the shift in perspective taking place. The bewitched perverts the dynamic social order and equates it with something as static as a law. The norm of solidarity and the gift become an obligation which it is impossible to conform to. I encountered the seeds of this discursive register in the interviews I conducted during the last six months of my fieldwork, at the homes of several elders in the village of Wanzamiso. When asked to talk about a general reality such as the community (rather than about specific persons), their replies were structured by the dualism of two desires common to all and hard to reconcile: bringing together (-*sanja*) and satiation (-*doshi*).

> Among people, in our Sukuma culture, what can cause you to become ill is when you start possessing things. That brings trouble, because you have overshadowed them. Many will stop liking you. I have seen it myself, and as far as hearing, I heard it all right. Your own kind, when you surpass them, they may list you as self-conceited: 'That one is full of himself'. And your family may stop liking you because of the wealth: 'He is self-conceited. That guy comes here. Hey, he is coming over, what should he eat? His type of food cannot be found here. "So, you people, what do you have?" He is too full of himself!'[1]

Sukuma typically criticize group processes such as rumours and false accusations, however, without denying the group's envy a moral basis. (In this discussion the difference between envy and jealousy seems inconsequential.) The arrogance of *ndoshi* comes with satiation, something undermining the commensality that people hold so dearly. However prone to illicit desires and extreme reactions, the witch manifests a judgement already latent in the group. Nobody can hope to please the *ndoshi*, to possess anything they may crave. Anyone who fears being labelled *ndoshi*, 'full of themselves', fears being seen as a person undermining the subtle exchange of hospitality and gift that preoccupies others. The educated Tanzanians of the development project I worked with, concluded from such conversations about *ndoshi* that they were fighting a war with development-resistant villagers who disliked the very things they in town promoted: economic progress and a change of lifestyle such as, quite typically, the building of durable houses roofed with corrugated iron sheets (*mabati*). I objected that the social distinction, profit and change promoted by the project were not incompatible with community values. The only problem was that they were couched in hierarchical terms that replaced the existing forms of social exchange.

The following words were spoken by a man who to me seemed quite representative of his fellow villagers, but referred to extreme interpretations, secretly put into practice by witches in the community.

> How do people know that you are full of yourself? For them it suffices that you have stopped suffering, or that you have built a nice house or a roof of corrugated iron sheets, then they will put you on the *ndoshi* side…. 'Where

does he sleep? He sleeps in there, that guy'.... Perhaps you are absent, or you don't stop by them, or you didn't do something for them, or maybe it is something you said? That is how they themselves speak to each other.

The label of self-conceit is brought in when you are not burdened by anything. The poor one will not be called *ndoshi*.... He will just be called one of the poor. What could he be possessing, whom could he fool? But you, if you have wealth, just utter a word ... one will say: 'Have you not seen that, so arrogant'.[2]

The verb repeatedly denoting the social position of the *ndoshi* is *ku-(ba)kila*, 'to surpass (them)'. Since the *ndoshi* does not transgress any rule, and the envious cannot claim any moral authority on their part, the tension lingers on in secrecy and anonymity. I asked an elder who was talking about gossip in the neighbourhood whether gossip led to isolation. 'No', he replied, 'you will go and visit people but fear is in your soul.... Mister, I should tell you, if you are being spoken of as *ndoshi*, then your life has shrunk. Your entire household gets into trouble'.[3] Here, excess of social pressure is expressed by a life 'shrinking' (*ku-geeha*), the opposite of 'being with' and self-expansion (*lukumo*, 'collection'). It is the lively social order shrinking to a deadening law. The duality of *busanja* (togetherness) and *budoshi* (complacency; *ndoshi* and *ku-dosa* are derivatives from the same stem) refers to the well-known difficult balance between the desire to be accepted by the group and the longing for self-assertion. Initiation, alliance and medicinal practice express this tension in terms of *kaya* (the homestead of the extended family) and *bu* (forest). *Busanja* refers to the reciprocity between home and forest, inside and outside, openness towards the other and mutual attraction. *Bugota*, 'medicine', exemplifies the reciprocity of home and forest, individual and group, celebrated in initiatory societies.

Brandström (1991) has described the ideology of domesticating the wild: Sukuma men identify with the patrilineage (*buta*) and the bow, an instrument of subjection held in the left hand, while women and the matrilineage are referred to as *ngongo*, 'the back', associated with the bare, natural force of the right hand. In this ideology the vital sources to be domesticated include cattle, women and unrelated families (with whom alliances are formed through marriage); the dead (propitiated through sacrifice); healing powers and the forest (mastered through initiation); and uncultivated terrain (cleared and cultivated with fire and hoe). We notice the reciprocity logic of the gift. The idea holds as well for the rains falling from the sky, via the 'king' (*ntemi*) who has always been situated outside the social order of daily life and who bears in him the signs of the wild, symbolizing the land itself (Tcherkézoff 1983). The 'unbounded universe' and logic of expansion, evocatively portrayed by Brandström, is an optimistic, yet vulnerable philosophy of life. The metaphor about an individual's life 'contracting' within the group illustrates this. The study of witchcraft continues from there.

The potential for something as foreboding as moral power is always present. A perilous moment in the gift dynamic is when a poor covillager or kin member requests a gift one is not willing to give. The vast literature on the 'evil eye' in North Africa and the Mediterranean treats this tension as arising when a beggar offers to cast away the evil eye in return for a small donation, or else the evil lingers. I once observed my friend Mashala dealing with this kind of social stress by ingeniously playing on the duality of *doshi* and *sanja*. To a younger cousin hoping to get some money, Mashala jokingly sighed: 'Oh, my cousin, don't you know that here at my place you have come to the house of Masanja's son, who maybe should return altogether to the *badoshi* back home at his father's place'. The father of Mashala is not called Masanja in real life. The name's literal meaning, derived from -*sanja* (bringing together), is telling enough, an epithet cherished by prosperous men. Masanja is the name given to children born in a period of good harvest. The son of Masanja, then, alludes to Mayala, 'hunger', because a year of hunger is supposed to succeed times of plenty. (The logic resembles that of the alternation of respect and joking between adjacent generations in greeting procedures.) What caused hilarity among those hearing the joke was the suggestion that in Masanja's homestead reigns *budoshi*. Everybody recognizes the ambivalence of clan relations. To parents and kin in general one cannot make gifts in the strict sense, because a blood tie, as it is given by birth, rules out the need of reciprocal giving. Kinship relations are governed by other principles, such as duty, privilege and help. (By analogy, development workers seeking to 'help' are behaving like kin, no matter how distant, and therefore better not expect anything in return, such as precious 'accountability'.) Son and daughter do not count the hours they worked for the family, herding cattle or performing household tasks. Nor does the father grant his sons a number of cattle as bridewealth proportional to the labour they have taken on. From this brief scene sliced from daily life we learn about the social stress arising at a kin member's request as well as how a complex of strategies can manage that stress. While alluding to his own poverty, Mashala had projected *budoshi* onto his parental generation, as well as recalled that kin relations are not ruled by the gift's cycle of debt and credit. He thus expertly avoided seeming like an *ndoshi* while undercutting his cousin's potential for moral power. His reaction was worthy of the initiated, matching forest and home.

Social status (*lukumo*) goes together with ancestral blessing (*lubango*). As in *ihane* initiation, the risky movement from the home (*kaya*) to the forest (*bu*) and back empowers the home and bolsters fertility. A number of Sukuma terms regarding the (variable) state of the world thus enter into one scheme, which contrasts the coolness of social exchange (<=>) with the heat of satiation or self-conceitedness, blurring the distinction between home and forest (=).

| | |
|---|---|
| *busanja* | *ndoshi* |
| *Kaya* <=> *Bu* | *Kaya* = *Bu* |
| *mhola* (cool) | *nsebu* (hot) |

Figure 5.1: Sukuma concepts of states of the world

# Culture and Experience

Chapter 3 introduced the 'cool' balance between gift and sacrifice, exemplified by initiations and by the magical potions drawn from the forest. Here we move on to the discursive register of 'heat', which is opposed to 'coolness' and in this sense is implied by it, albeit negatively. The witch is 'hot' because she perverts the exchange between inside and outside. The use of local terminology and of interview fragments might reinforce the impression that we are approximating the local perspective, people's 'philosophy of life' so to speak. But local opinions and local terms offer no guarantee for understanding their meaning. Remember my neighbour talking of levelling pressures and of something quite different as well: his defiance of these pressures. Why would it seem to us that he is contradicting himself? A decisive moment in my analysis is to face the danger of a legalistic concept of culture. Take the example of *ihane* novices. They were said to make themselves 'hot'. Since they were intruders, becoming 'a forest from within the home' and entitled to carry the magical bundle *bu ya mu kaya*, our analysis would lead us to infer that they became witches. However, they were not, as I demonstrated, because something external and variable mediated the meaning of culture, its practices and beliefs. It is called experience.

Social scientists are classically inclined to a legalistic understanding of culture. They treat culture as an internalized programme, a set of dispositions or 'habitus' (however 'dynamic' and 'versatile') on the basis of which individuals act, for example in interaction with the environment and 'social field' (see Bourdieu 1980). From the data we should more or less predict what 'the Sukuma' will experience and do. The trouble with this view of culture is that it conflates experiencing and doing, as if the only interaction that students of culture should consider is the social one between an individual's dispositions to act and the changing environment. Experience, a structuring of the world, comes in between. Culture determines experience. But the inverse influence is true as well. This means that we must be willing to consider the part in experience that is independent from culture; or, better still, the part that determines culture rather than is determined by culture. Why are the intruders who bring the 'forest' within the 'home' not witches? The answer is the experiential structure of initiation. Its tenor is flexible and reciprocal. In a frame of experience that is rigid and intrusive, the novices would come across as witches. Within that frame, people with certain features (such as 'red eyes', 'elderly' and 'female', to name a few of the traits often selected) will always be suspect. Like the bewitched, students of culture are at risk from applying this rigid and intrusive frame.

How come anthropologists tend to neglect the role of experiential shifts when they determine the meaning of cultural data? How come, for example, they treat witchcraft as a practice and the witch as an actor, even if both are locally treated as being of hypothetical status? (A Sukuma diviner exclaiming 'Witches really do exist, you know!' in my view underlines that status.) Perhaps modern reason has the predilection to present itself as frameless. Perhaps our Judeo-Christian dichotomy of good and evil fails to grasp how Sukuma could on the one hand despise witches and on the other hand boast about their own powerful magic (not to speak of their ease in negotiating rules, whose violations are forgotten after a fine is paid). The next section shows that a legalistic understanding of culture in the study of witchcraft has absurd consequences. If suspecting the paternal aunt of witchcraft (a common pattern of accusation among Sukuma) did not stem from the particular frame in which the victim experiences and reconstructs the world, but were a socialized belief about the witch's identity, hence of identical status to a factual discovery, then – I can hardly contain the exclamation mark – there would simply be no paternal aunts left by now.

Clearly, we cannot avoid the experiential issue in the study of culture. It is not a matter of diversity or volatility or even multilayered-ness, as is so often claimed about culture. Experience brings in a culture's fundamental and recurring shifts between opposite positions. Development projects proclaim that their proposals are 'culture-sensitive' if accepted by consensus in the community, for instance in the context of a 'participatory rural appraisal' (PRA) in which villagers define problems in dialogue with NGO experts. 'Let the people decide' is an excuse to avoid the comparative exercise of studying a culture. Culture is not equivalent to a PRA consensus or the sum total of answers obtained from a survey and interviews. Ask any number of Sukuma (or Belgians) whether they want to be given the material benefits an NGO has to offer: the high score that is more than likely obtained tells you less about the culture than about the new situation caused by the question. Culture is particular to a group, but none of its members (or their sum) possesses it in conveyable form. At the same time, the only conveyable form a culture can take, as in these pages, is that of an individual experience. Although expressed in socially formed and culturally specific terms, it refers to a human reality, which is not particular to one culture. That is the point of experiential structures. I hope this will become clear, as we reach this pivotal moment and return to Lukundula's compound to investigate the situation generating a particular construct of the witch.

# The Pure Reason of the Witch

How sensations of pain and intrusion, often articulated as poisoning, could grow into an embodied, concrete idea about the hatred and envy of one's near kin, I observed during my work with Sukuma healers and their patients. They confronted me with a curious paradox about the face of evil. Going by the more than fifty cases of witchcraft I studied, the relation between witch and victim is one of intimacy, intrusion and absolute debt. Patients regularly and spontaneously spoke of the witch's motive, namely her judgement of them as complacent, *badoshi*. The witch had seen them think: 'What do you have that I may need?' The paradox is that patients allege that they deserve their illness. They subsume the witch's grudge under the same category as the ancestor's anger. The ancestral spirit, *isamva*, a term I translate literally as 'the provoked one' (from –*samba*, to provoke), brings illness when provoked by the descendant's neglect. The ancestor might be entitled to anger. Remarkably, the witch too executes the arrogant, who have violated the social law strictly defined. She punishes them with death for evading the gift system, for denying others the attention and respect that comes with social exchange. Contrary to the typical picture of an outcast at the periphery of society, the witch should be located at the heart of society, if in its deepest, invisible core. The witch has moral power.

A genealogical survey conducted in 1997 by one of my Sukuma collaborators, Ndaki Munyeti, seems to confirm this moral aspect of the witch. Of 77 household heads interviewed, only one third were willing to point out suspected witches and their respective victims on their family tree, so the results are indicative, merely lending support to the more revealing qualitative data cited below.[4] But it was remarkable to see the invisible network of witchcraft relations rise from these genealogies. The 25 family trees contained 81 cases of fatal witchcraft attributed to 38 suspects in total. The victims were men and women (48 versus 33). One would expect the suspects to be evenly spread too, but they weren't. The witches were almost all female, with just one male witch, a childless man whose victim was a fertile brother. Three kinship positions in relation to the victim topped our survey: the paternal grandmother (12 out of 38 suspects; 25 out of 81 cases), the coresident sister-in-law (9 out of 38 suspects; 16 out of 81 cases) and the paternal aunt (6 out of 38 suspects; 14 out of 81 cases). The other 11 suspected witches were evenly divided between mother, wife, sister and great-grandmother. We noticed that the three most common kinship positions all related to the victim as an outsider within: all three combine insidership (as kin or living in) with the impregnable features of an outsider to the gift system, not or no longer available for marriage.

A classic riddle no Sukuma fails to solve hints at the role of the (paternal) grandmother: Grandmother with the broad back? The attic! (*Maama ngongo ngali? Likano!*). The attic (*likano*) was traditionally built above the inner, circular room of the house, where calves and small livestock were kept overnight. In the attic, certain foodstuffs and medicines are stored or hung from the roof. Inside the house and yet concealed, as well as covering the inhabitants, the attic bears resemblance to the grandmother and her 'broad back'. She takes care of the kitchen, the food supplies and some of the medicinal herbs, which means that besides controlling people's intake of foreign matter into the body, she is more inwardly located in the homestead than anyone else, despite coming from a foreign clan. We notice again that inside and outside, the two poles necessary for exchange, are combined in this outsider within. For men, the elderly woman's absolute outsidership consists in her impregnable position; she is barren and no potential candidate for marriage, alliance or other forms of social exchange.[5] But the paternal grandmother is an insider as well. As the eldest wife she performed the ritual of 'arranging the cooking space' (*kuhigika mahiga*) whereby she moved in all her cooking utensils and put her three hearthstones in place. At two occasions of serious crisis I have seen this spell being ritually expelled by the household head and his younger brother. They assailed this female space, extinguished the kitchen fire by using a bundle of leaves to sprinkle a protective liquid over it, replaced the hearthstones, and rekindled its fire in the traditional way.

The link between the elderly woman and the witch can be found in many cultures across the world. Inferring from this that elderly ladies are despised in those cultures is the error I have been trying to avoid. Rather than speaking of witchcraft in terms of static customs and beliefs, we should account for bewitchment. Bewitchment stands for a temporal experience producing a temporal association, whereby a particular member of the subject's social network coalesces with the above structural position of intrusion.

To unravel this generative process, I find the interviews I had with healers are very helpful. Looking back on their careers, many mentioned as the primordial witch the victim's paternal aunt (*sengi*), the third most common suspect in the above survey. The explanation they gave to me was that she secretly demanded 'the cattle of her lap' (*ng'ombe ja matango gakwe*). This condensed metaphor suggests that the paternal aunt makes a sacrifice at marriage by moving out of her family in return for a large number of cattle. The cattle from her now impoverished in-laws later allow her brother to marry with bridewealth and have his children belong to the clan with all the social status that comes with this. The reasoning is that harm to those children – in the form of illness, misfortune or death – would compensate for their aunt's sacrifice. The sinister demand for 'the cattle of my lap' imputes to the paternal aunt the following reasoning: 'I sacrificed myself, went to live at another family where I had to work hard to make up for the cattle they lost because of me, only to realize that, when push comes to shove, my children are not my children but belong to my husband's clan. And thanks to me my brothers have children. Well, this is unfair. Following the logic of the gift I am entitled to the lives of my brothers' children'. The *ng'winga*, 'the one who left,' as every bride is called, gets back at the *ndoshi* back home. That is the reason – as in both 'the reasoning' and 'the motive' – of the witch.

Or, at least, that is the reasoning imputed to the paternal aunt by those suspecting her. Let us follow the example of the healers. What they did by explaining to me people's primordial suspicion is to introduce experiential frames. Once we do this, we trace behind the reason of the witch the reasoning of the one who invents her, the victim. More exactly, we observe the product of a socially and experientially formed frame of powerlessness. The crux of my analysis is that in terms of the Sukuma balance of gift and sacrifice this concrete expression of a person's bewitchment is absurd. The construct of the paternal aunt as witch requires us to think away the Sukuma custom that distinguishes gift and sacrifice. We know from the previous chapter that the logic of the gift, whereby high debts (*shili* from the verb *kulya*, 'to eat') socially 'eat' a person, should not apply to relations with paternal aunts. The aunt takes no credit for her marital transaction as she merely did a bride's duty. The crucial point, then, is that bewitchment changes things. It breaks with tradition, indicating (as argued below) that the bewitched spontaneously purify reason in a way we moderns do. How else could one speculate on an aunt's claim to compensation for bridewealth? I see no other explanation: rather than a contradiction in Sukuma culture, we are observing an experiential shift.

135

The interdependence of gift and sacrifice is too 'peaceful' or 'cool' a condition of the world to be of any relevance to the bewitched, in this case patients suffering from affliction, expecting to die, or mourning the loss of beloved ones. Their experience alters culture at those (exceptional) moments. What has hampered anthropology in the past has been the emphasis on the other direction of influence; that is, culture – in the form of belief in the paternal aunt as witch, for example – determines experience.

In constructing the paternal aunt as witch, the frames of gift and sacrifice are temporarily conflated, their cherished magical interrelation suspended. The paternal aunt's sacrifice is reinterpreted in terms of a gift. If a sacrifice that supports the whole system of the gift enters that very system, what will be the result? A bottomless debt. Nothing else could so well express the victim's experience. The very person who incarnates the medium of the gift system and could not be domesticated by the system, now intrudes the system. This is what suspecting the paternal aunt means. The victims apply the social law in a perversely purified manner, deeming the transaction of their life (or that of beloved ones) as a genuine possibility. Figure 5.2 schematizes this construction of the witch. True to the purity of the victim's crisis, a life has to be traded for a life.

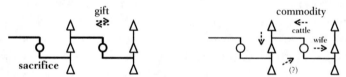

Figure 5.2: Bewitchment as experiential shift: from gift/sacrifice to commodity

Bewitchment represents an experiential shift, from the magical balance of gift and sacrifice to their conflation in the logic of commoditization. Figure 5.2 depicts on the left the traditional distinction, and alternation, between relations of sacrifice within the clan (bold lines) and relations of gift ruling the exchange between clans through women and bridewealth (in the figure: clan <=> clan). The right half of the figure depicts the view of the bewitched. The traditional distinction of gift and sacrifice has vanished (no bold lines). As a result, the one logic ruling social exchange is that of commodity transaction. In kinship terms the right half of the figure pictures a paternal aunt entering a closed system, a gloomy cycle where a wife is interchangeable with the cattle handed down to her brother, and those cattle are in turn interchangeable with her brother's child. The witch's circle is rounded with the paternal aunt's initial 'gift' returning in the form of a person's life (the question mark).

As in any shift, it is necessary to know the point of departure. The ethnography showed this point to be the magical balance of gift and sacrifice. In our earlier formula (see Figure 4.2), this point is the $e$ on which the meaning of $p$ depends. Until now anthropologists have not considered $e$, assuming that this basic structure of experience is the same for all humans. Cultural symbolics and identities are what would be plural (excessively plural since they would have no experiential layer of connection). By keeping $e$ constant (using the positivist fiction of 'all things being equal', *ceteris paribus*) they universalized the $e1$ of positivism, the action and reaction of formal logic, of Aristotle's law of the excluded third. Anthropology, the one discipline meant to explore other cultures, has been too prejudiced about magic to discuss meaning from magic's perspective ($e2$). Stronger still, anthropology privileged one particular frame ($e1$), that of modern pure reason. It happens to be that of the bewitched, those inventing the witch, who rationalize magic and thus, we will see, are liable to resort to the machete instead of counter-magic and ritual.

The bewitched purify social exchange. What remains is the law, the calculus of debt and credit. The table of social exchange, Figure 4.1, equated this logic with that of the first column: commodities (purified gifts). The witch arises from commodity logic. The immoral traits often claimed publicly about the witch conceal a hyper-moral figure. The witch reinforces the law. She impairs metacommunicative frames, as I argued when comparing Bateson's and Lacan's theory of schizophrenia in Chapter 2: patients of *mayabu* bewitchment suffer from the excluded third (or father). They suffer from positivism, from commodity logic – a morality in its own right, in fact the harshest kind. The victim becomes, as Sukuma say, a zombie, *litunga* (from *ku-tunga*), literally 'tied' to the witch. Crisis sparks off devastating moral power, as attested to by the social-sensory-experiential frame of intrusion. It is a morality that radically reduces people's experiential palette and 'contracts' their life. It is the purification that we earlier dubbed modern.

Remember Lemi standing in the centre of Seele's compound and professing resolutely 'I am Jesus!' His arms wide open and head slightly tilted backwards, he watched with fulfilment how his sudden pause affected us. It sent a shiver up my spine to imagine what these words meant for my Sukuma friends, who heard the witch talking. What better incarnation of moral power than Jesus, a saviour crucified? Lemi's condition of *mayabu* and screams of despair are the flesh-and-blood of moral power. His logorrhoea materializes the harsh, unnegotiable law circulating in the socio-economic system that he as a trader had become part of.

Remember Albert's finger pointing at his paternal aunt. Her jealousy over his successful receipt of cattle in return for his daughter echoes the predicament of the bride expressed in the wedding song. 'Liars!' she sings, while her family goes on about the custom since time immemorial of exchanging 'cattle and a person'. The song's insistence on where the logic of debts applies and where that of duty, is too conspicuous to maintain that traditions are so deeply socialized that no experience could undermine them. I learned that humans do not concur with their cultures. Thanks to the experiential angle, I could recognize more from Sukuma culture than socialization theorists predict, while the epistemological challenge to capture the culture was greater than ethnographic data suggest. I could not do without the comparative work, tentatively articulated in the formula, the table and this figure above (see Figures 4.1, 4.2 and 5.2).

Many suspects were not paternal aunts. Some, although few, were not absolute outsiders within. But the trend expressive of the frame of intrusion outlined here cannot be denied. Much of my ethnographic data tell of the peculiar kinship position of the paternal aunt. During initiation into the society of elders, her position featured in one of the metaphors conveyed. At the liminal stage when novices reach a state of 'heat' and their former selves die, they had a heavy stone hung around their neck by an elder who whispered '*Sengi!*', the paternal aunt. In a moment of creativity and a sensorily 'hot' state something essential was said to the initiated about the precariousness of tradition. I am aware that etymology itself is not evidence of meaning. But as one element among many converging ones, the verb that *sengi* probably stems from, is revealing: *ku–senga*, 'to clear the bush for a house', evokes the commencement of social life. By analogy, the bride's sacrifice allows her clan to participate in social exchange.

Witch constructs arise from experiential shifts, themselves effected by social conditions. Additional evidence is that the figure of intrusion persists even as the primordial witch changes. Sukuma elders told me that over the last three decades 'the *sengi* has been replaced by the neighbour'. The concept of insidership has changed, as the alluring distance between compounds disappeared due to increased population density as well as the villagization programme of Nyerere's *ujamaa* in the late 1970s. 'Faint odours of cooking reached the neighbour', while expectations of invitation could not be met. In the words of the elders, this gave cause for envy and witchcraft retaliation. 'On breaking up the *ujamaa* villages and returning to our separate plots, we saw what villagization had done. Graves of children were scattered all over the place'. Suspicion of witchcraft had increased and the list of suspects had expanded. An increase in affliction in the new villages came with more grounds to fear envy or reproach. As the centre of gravity veered from kinship to village community, the neighbour now too, no less than the paternal aunt did before, embodied moral power. The next section elaborates on this point, before continuing with our witchcraft analysis.

# From Polycentric to Monocentric

Sukuma appear to situate the experience that breeds witchcraft suspicions not in the fresh ambience of magic and wonder but in the festering, putrid atmosphere of disenchantment. This tendency of bewitchment coming after pleasure was often described to me. The following respondent reflects on recent seductions and 'our sweetness of the body' (*butamu wise bo mili*). The word 'sweetness', *butamu*, is derived from the Swahili adjective for sweet, *tamu*. He describes how the outsider, 'the hidden' (*misa*), can become a witch after having become an insider, such as an extra-marital partner. The period of 'growing population' refers to Nyerere's villagization programme in the mid 1970s.

> They [witches] started especially in the period of growing population, because then the outsider came along with the sweetness which we are made of. Both man and woman, each person has this desire, the sweetness of the body. So, the outsider could be invited at one's home. I go with her, she confides in me. I have gone with her and then I may change my mind, thinking that this woman actually does not satisfy me.... So, she sets up a conspiracy: 'Gee, so-and-so is really arrogant, I could only sleep once with him!' Thus a woman sets a trap.[6]

Population pressure became a visible fact after the villagization campaign called *operesheni vijijini* (operation at the villages). Hyden (1980), Abrahams (1987: 194ff), Brandström (1991), Waters (1997) and others have extensively dealt with this ambitious, modernizing endeavour, fostered by the planned economy and good intentions. They have assessed the programme's failure to anticipate the ill effects of relocation and the centralization of homesteads on agro-pastoral people like the Sukuma and Nyamwezi. Positively determined to provide education and healthcare for all citizens, the government forced farmers to move to artificially mapped villages, centred around a school and dispensary. Stragglers were spurred on, as traditional round houses of grass and clay – which undermined the nation's sweeping belief in *maendeleo* (the Swahili term for progress) – were set on fire. The whole operation turned out to be counterproductive for stock breeding as well as for the cultivation of staple crops, partly due to homesteads being separated from their fields and cattle, which hindered farmers giving them the attention they needed. Furthermore, the density of cattle produced by villagization resulted in land erosion and diminishing pasturage. When the failure of the programme became obvious, only a few years after its inception, most people started returning to their former lands, the so-called *mahame* (from the Swahili *ku-hama*, 'to emigrate').

However, when talking on an intimate basis with Sukuma elders about the villagization programme, none of the above observations were prominent. Were they too obvious? Or is it because considerations sprang to mind that were considered to be more important? Elders claimed that, most of all, villagization had boosted the practice of witchcraft in the community – or at least had increased suspicions and accusations of that kind.[7] It is generally felt that witchcraft occurs more than ever before. Furthermore, I was told that formerly people would primarily fear their kin, but since villagization and the subsequent return to former lands the belief began to spread that virtually everybody, starting from your neighbours, could be a witch.

What could be the reason for this double observation, of more witchcraft and an unbounded extension of the list of potential witches? Macro-sociological explanations of the kind Tanner (1970) has offered for Sukuma witch-hunts prior to the 1970s suggest higher social density produces an increased chance of conflict arising between neighbours. Furthermore, Simeon Mesaki (1994: 55ff) points out that Sukumaland would seem to support Mary Douglas's argument linking witchcraft beliefs to small-scale, densely populated, sedentary groupings with a high dynamic density of interaction and internal competition. But do such densely populated communities in Africa always experience more sorcery than others? And can such a general explanation account for the Sukuma case, more particularly for the cultural patterns of witch construction? This debate brings us back to the impressive enterprise of structural-functionalist research undertaken by Gluckman (1970), Marwick (1970) and others, where sorcery is explained in terms of social conflicts generated by contradictions in the social and normative order of communities. In the case of the Sukuma and Nyamwezi, Abrahams (1994: 15ff) has added the political dimension to the debate: by analogy with the rise of Sungusungu vigilante groups, witch killings can be understood in the context of disappearing chieftainship and the limited local relevance of the national government, which have together impelled villagers to rely on their own resources of action.

Far from contesting these assertions, I would argue that while socio-structural processes, historical changes and government policies are enacted, the core of the matter remains that when Sukuma fall seriously ill – and people continue to do so – they usually attribute the cause to someone bewitching them. Instead of denouncing functionalist or macro-sociological theories on the basis of their alleged unfashionable status, I point to the experiential basis these theories lack. I prefer the intuitive track of reasoning proposed by Sukuma themselves. What happened during villagization when each house neighboured another? One elder tried to explain this to me in the following words:

> Now your neighbours could see every day how your wife was preparing a fish for a nice meal, but you couldn't invite them. This situation, you may expect that it makes your neighbours jealous. They may think to themselves: '*Wadosile sana*, you feel you're too good for me. Well, you will see...'

Fish and the Swahili word *sana* – in the expression *Wadosile sana* ('You are very arrogant') – pop up in these accounts, invoking the imagery of alleged promiscuity, arrogance and undeserved fortune that are associated with the lakeshore fishermen and Swahili-speaking towns. Others tell of feelings of reproach for not greeting

141

neighbours properly. 'You will see' leaves little room for speculation as to the outcome hinted at.

> When we rejoined the *ujamaa* village, we built all right. When we came to the village, we were afraid of each other. We were still very Sukuma in those beginnings. You would wait until the other greets you first... There was anxiety of the kind: 'If I do not greet him, I will be told so'. Anyway, we saw that urge wearing out. Acceptance came in: perhaps you know him [enough to greet] but you don't care. You're surprised? This villagization was problematic! Anyway, when moving out with our families from [names of villages], we discovered graves scattered everywhere. Of small children, each homestead.[8]

This man voices the mainstream opinion on the government's settlement policy. The surge of suspicion corresponded to the centralization of households, because the latter implied a radical shift in the spatial sphere and thus of social relations. To replace the polycentric landscape by a monocentric or village-type of spatial order put heavy pressures on Sukuma society. To put it cynically, who would have thought that Sukuma had a culture and that culture could be more than an arbitrary set of beliefs? Not even development anthropologists can get used to the idea that cultures could actually have been meticulously built up by the group through trial and error to serve collective well-being with no single member able to speak for this process or replace it.

The boundaries and ensuing interactions between interior and exterior were undercut as the fence between them was brought down and the mediation-prone distance that separated households shrivelled away. Households were suddenly confronted with each other without being able to comply with the unspoken law of society that prescribes social exchange between independent homes. This social law has been translated in the Sukuma norm of hospitality, where copresence or sharing a place necessarily entails sharing food and speech. In this new situation of spatial density neighbours were prevented from consistently following their urge to reciprocate as eyes meet. The alternative would have been to invite each other daily and thus to absorb one another in a sort of aimless potlatch. In short, the spatial shift placed people in the structural position of acting like *badoshi*. They were involuntarily attesting to a negligent or conceited attitude. And they could not avoid the neighbour's feeling of deprivation for lack of the Sukuma's well-tried method of dissolving envy though greeting and other kinds of social exchange.

But is the lack of social exchange sufficient for neighbours to poison each other? In ethnographic accounts prior to the villagization program (e.g., Tanner 1970), we can read that even then accusations and witch killings were not limited to the extended family or kin group but involved the larger community. The elders' remarks that formerly only your kin would be suspected does not hint at a Sukuma maxim but stresses the sharp contrast with the situation prior to the mid 1970s. Villagization was an acceleration of the modernization already taking place. Outsiders occupied positions comparable to that of an insider, as they were privy to daily life in the neighbouring homestead. Since the witch has to know you, your activities and the names of your ancestors, the list of potential bearers of a grudge with the ability to put spite into practice radically expanded.

# Opposite Structures of Experience

What does it mean for anyone to label the paternal aunt as the primordial witch? One could easily overlook the theoretical implication. Ethnographers might think that they have established a cultural belief, a belief that, if socialized well, should determine experience and practice. Yet no Sukuma showed trepidation in greeting paternal aunts or in having them stay over. Given the collective aversion to the witch, and given that about every woman is a paternal aunt to someone, we could expect Sukuma to be hunting down these family members and potential witches, with the result that all Sukuma women should have been eliminated by now. We recognize the absurdity of considering culture without experience. Cultural beliefs only matter to the extent that they partake of situations; that they are structured, emplaced. Situations are, of course, as much social as they are cognitive or biological. Two examples of situations where the ominous quality of *sengi* come to the fore are the healer's compound and the creative mood during ritual at the point of the novice's virtual death.

Absurdities following the abstraction and removal of experience from culture have plagued anthropology since functionalism. To state that social change and competition over new goods increase witchcraft suspicions (e.g., Marwick 1952: 129; Mitchell 1956) hardly accords with the reality on the ground, where suspicion is pointless without an actual experience of illness first. Fierce competition yielding wealth and good health need not raise the possibility of witchcraft; a stable society in which an epidemic has broken out will more probably lead to a great deal of witchcraft accusation. Culture is not a collection of axioms members are bound by, irrespective of their experience. In functionalist studies every culture was supposed to have its fixed scapegoat or 'fifth colonne' (Middleton 1963; Marwick 1970; see also Girard 1993). Gluckman (1970: 224) learned from his Zulu informants that women 'have evil in their nature' while men employ magic openly and legitimately. My data about the Sukuma paternal aunt could have been misread as another such axiom, had we not looked at the experiential frames of the belief, and the shifts between these.

Consider the following remarks of Middleton, writing about the Lugbara of Uganda: 'A man who is bewitched is held partly to blame for it. If he were not rude or insolent to someone else, he would not arouse the other's anger or possibly his power of witchcraft,' a statement which is subsequently contradicted: 'witches are axiomatically evil people, so that the victim cannot be blamed' (Middleton 1963: 272). Now, include the experiential shift and the contradiction vanishes at the spot. What Middleton registered was at one moment Lugbara victims privately recounting their suspicions and at another the public discourse of those feeling strong enough to accuse. Witchcraft studies of the process of accusation and rumour highlight an important side of the phenomenon (Stewart and Strathern 2004; Siegel 2006), but it is only one side. True, a patient has several paternal aunts; and it is possible that the one accused previously by others is more likely to be suspected. But these concrete factors of influence reveal little about the process of suspicion. Accusations are often strategic. Turner (1968) described how Ndembu solved the contradiction between virilocal residence and matrilineal kinship burdening their society. They accused their in-laws of witchcraft in order to break up their daughter's marriage and get her children to come over and live with her matrilineage. Yet, accusations and other power strategies reveal nothing about the witch someone really suspects. An experience of powerlessness is not an experience of less power. Powerlessness belongs to another frame altogether. So too do suspicions. To be able to accuse, the patient has to first complete a transformation, often at the healer's place and after divination that brings to light suspicions sometimes so deeply disturbing they smother all meaningful speech. Only then do patients cast away the imagery of a moral Other entitled to their life and dare to speak up and assert themselves; that is, enter the frame of accusation and counter-magic.

The distinction and shift between experiential frames, essential to Sukuma healing as I will argue, is lacking in Favret-Saada's (1980) description of witchcraft and healing in the Bocage, France. She holds that the life-forces of sorcerer, patient and healer are engaged in a magical battle, whereby healers ('strong force') replace patients ('weak force') in order to fight the sorcerers, who lose their strong position and become weak like the patients were before (ibid.: 95ff). I will show that this magical exchange, staging a reciprocal battle with the 'witch', is only the endpoint of a therapeutic process which begins with the very different attempt of breaking the spell of disempowerment. The victim experiences the moral power of an Other, an absolute outsider within. In divination and magic the 'Other' retreats to be replaced by an opponent or particular other (without capital 'O'). Favret-Saada's concept of 'force' (ibid.: 251), a vital energy inhabiting people and circulating among them, occludes the existential breach between self and other which Seele's patients shared with us.

The clear pattern in gender and kinship position of the paternal aunt may fool ethnographers into taking the witch's identity for a socialized belief rather than for an experience spontaneously formed in response to a social situation. If we keep the experiential factor constant, we can expect the category of witch to include major users of magic such as the chief, dancer or members of some cult (like the Wicca in Europe). But anthropologists speaking of such concrete others as witches and discussing their 'craft' (Luhrman 1989) are dealing with another experiential structure than that of victims constructing their witch. Most Sukuma employ magical recipes, we have seen. 'Aren't we all witches?' the bartender asked. Magic establishes reciprocity with the natural and social environment. The proverbial dancer does not hold a secretive grudge. No user of magic identifies with the witch's envy and moralism. The frame of magic is entirely at odds with that of witch construction.

The analytical neglect of experiential frames has resulted in conflation, hence contradiction. Geschiere (1997: 24) noticed the contradictions but attributed them to the ambiguity of witchcraft. What we have differentiated as the frames of accusation (power) and suspicion (powerlessness) appear in his analysis as two 'forces' of witchcraft, accumulative and levelling. Extending Bayart's (1993) thesis on 'the politics of the belly', Geschiere describes the African chief boasting about his magical powers to eliminate rivals and accumulate capital. At the same time, Geschiere (1997: 77) insists on the secrecy surrounding the topic and the difficulty of getting information, since nobody likes to be associated with the bewitchment of kin out of envy. He thus switches to the witchcraft a chief, politician or dancer will not readily be suspected of, let alone boast about. Much like Middleton on the Lugbara, Geschiere stumbles onto frames of experience but treats them as equivalent elements of a culture, ignoring their opposition and the shift between them. Karp (1980: 96, 111) likewise records that Iteso in Kenya defined the witch as 'a-social'. Young students visiting their home village were seen as a-social. But in the actual cases studied by Karp the reader notices that, contrary to the logical deduction, students were not suspected of inflicting harm. The fact that their success causes jealousy clears them of suspicion and actually makes them likely victims.

Kapferer's (1997: 17, 262) invaluable study of Sinhalese sorcery brings out the cosmology of agency, destruction and creation that underlies the use of magic. That same cosmology shines through in the deep conviction proper to witchcraft beliefs that harm must have its origin in the agency of people. Yet, as I have argued, more than one cosmological frame is at work in the healer's compound. The agency of rich immigrants intrudes upon the community, raising questions as to the magical means they have adopted for their success and thus making them an easy target for collective accusation. But surely they are the last to be suspected of jealousy. The cosmology of creative force ('unreason', see Kapferer 2003) has allured anthropologists and will illuminate our study of ritual, but for witchcraft we must comprehend its opposite, the cosmology of pure reason. The ritual celebration of human agency and the secret act born of jealousy are opposite motives. Magic and bewitchment tap into different states of the system.

The ambiguity (from the Latin *ambi*, 'both ways', and *agere*, 'driving') of witchcraft springs from the fusion of two opposite frames of experience. The object of attack will experience (and reinvent) witchcraft differently from the user of magic. The ethnography permits one to tell sorcery and bewitchment apart, to shift attention from the witch's craft to the witch's reason. Little insight in the experiential shift can be expected from describing magical practices alone (the frame of power) as Malinowski (1922) did. Evans-Pritchard (1976) too approached the witch as an actor. His Azande informants distinguished the conscious application of 'sorcery' from the unconscious inner evil called 'witchcraft'. The latter, witches proper, cannot be interviewed about this inner action, for they know nothing about it. The anthropologist's job, it seems to me, is not to support or verify the Zande hypothesis, but to describe it and, by way of analysis, relate it contextually. We study where an idea comes from (versus whether it is true or not). This is what I mean by the frame of experience. Then we discern in the sorcerer and the witch not two types of action or two kinds of actor but two products of cultural creativity. We ask how these concepts may stem from distinct experiences of the world, perhaps shifting between the frame of power (public magical competition) and the frame of powerlessness (impulsive secretive intrusions).

Why has acknowledging frames, their opposition and shift, not been an obvious thing in anthropology? Shifts in experience refer to events, while the Cartesian divide of nature and culture locates meaning in a culture conceived as a synchronic network of signifiers. To state something about 'a' culture, many scholars feel they need to disregard natural events and consequently elide the experiential as 'all things being equal'.

Underlying the frames is a moral issue. Seele's patients hated the witch to the point of wishing her dead. Yet, evil as in illicit behaviour sheds no light on the witch of their making. Sukuma conceive of social exchange dynamically enough to accept transgressions as part of life. Magic is part of their dance competitions, and of the continuous destabilization of social law through sacrificial logic. So we need to look beyond the dualism of good and evil. Therefore I have situated the logic of the bewitched within a quaternary, holistic structure of social exchange. If witchcraft is the dark side of social exchange (Godbout 1992) and we define social exchange in this dynamic way, then this 'dark side' can be imagined to have the opposite quality of dynamic. The utterly static is precisely what I mean by pure reason and by the hyper-social moralism of the witch's power. The sensuously wild and asocial transgressions recounted in urban legends have been misleading us. They have tempted studies of witchcraft into reproducing the exotic, occult Africa dreamt up by our colonial ancestors. Something much more recognizable and universal is at issue.

On this basis we may answer Kapferer's (1997: 17) question about the widespread association of the witch's reason with envy. Merleau-Ponty defined envy as the non-differentiation of I and other (cited in Grosz 1990: 42). Envy does not invert but pervert the Sukuma value of communal solidarity, for it treats I and other as non-different, equal, so much so that anybody excluded from good fortune is entitled to be jealous and to bewitch.[9] The Sukuma synonym for witch (*nogi*) is the compound noun *ng'wiboneeji*, whose morphemes convey a profound message. Based on the linguistic formulas of derivation applied to the Sukuma language (see Richardson 1966: 9; Batibo 1985: 166, 171) the word can be split into its stem 'to see' (-*bon-*), the reflexive prefix (*i-*), the causative suffix (-*y*) and the amplifying suffix (-*eela*). The literal translation of *ng'wiboneeji* strikes me as remarkably significant in terms of our argument: 'the one who causes to see oneself persistently'.[10]

Although it is doubtful that my Sukuma friends experienced the word in this literal way, I can think of no better definition of moral power. The 'causing to see' reminds one of Levinas's morality of the other's gaze, but the persistence alludes to morality in the extreme, which is what I understand by moral power. Another person's moralizing (rather than moral) presence: is that not the claim of 'the cattle of her lap' imputed to the paternal aunt's silent stare? Is that not the neighbour's gaze in the monocentric villages imposed during the State's villagization programme? The structure of bewitchment explains why Tanzania's take on modernity has been a villagization policy placing Sukuma farmers in an inferior position and the national government (not unlike the Church) in a non-reciprocal position of correctness.

The semantic structure of *ng'wiboneeji* is not clear on whether the witch persists in making her see herself (comparing herself to others and thus becoming jealous) or in making the victim see themselves (placing a mirror before them and thus pointing the finger). Both seem applicable. Most of my informants opted for the second meaning because of the related curse *ibona*, which refers to the witch's revenge: 'you will see'. Those who wronged her will 'see' themselves; that is, have their due, meet their fate. As explained in Chapter 2, the *ibona* curse belongs to the category of *ndagu*, a 'fate'.

The new wave of witchcraft studies in the 1980s and 1990s, with Bayart and Geschiere at the forefront, discerned a 'politics of the belly' in postcolonial Africa whereby rulers at various echelons of power acquitted themselves as sorcerers devouring others to expand their network and 'belly'. Mbembe's (2001) material collected from the media, the public political arena and its hidden scenes confirmed this occult figure of power. But witchcraft is more than power, I have argued. It is also about powerlessness, which is not 'less' or 'very little' power. It introduces a frame of its own. Data obtained from the healer's compound enlightens here. I have kept another telling bit of evidence until the end. Against 'the belly' preoccupying contemporary anthropologists, Sukuma patients point to 'the liver', something that does not pleasurably expand. The witch is said to act from a pang of jealousy called *kitema* (from -*tema*, 'to cut'). The impulse originates in the liver, itself named *itema*.[11] The liver makes an important contrast with the accumulation of power and status ('collection', *lukumo*) and indeed with the expansion of the 'belly' by the dancer, the chief or the expert in magic.

Feeling neglected induces *kitema*. The witch does not transgress the social law or subvert the social order, gratifying illicit desires. The witch rigidifies the law, transforming a dynamic into something purely static. Monica Wilson (1951: 313) was right not to indulge her audience and refer to a wet dream when famously defining the witch as the 'standardized nightmare' of a group.

# Notes

1. *Umu bamunhu, umu kisukuma shise ishikenhelejaga kubiza na nsaata amashikolo ulu ugapandika. Gakenhaga imilibanga nguno abiyo wabakija. Boya ukukutogwa abingi. Nagubona n'ung'wene, n'ukwigwa niigwa duhu. Abiyo angu, ulu ubakija, bukutuula ha budoshi: 'Wadosa ung'wenuyu'. Na abaduguyo boyaga ukukutogwa kulwa shikolo: 'Wadosa. Wiza henaha ung'wenuyu. Hi, aliiza, alye ki? Shitiho isha kulya ung'wene ahenaha. "Ning'we mulina ki?" Wadosa no!'*

2. *Bakukumana kinehe giki ubebe wadosa? Aboyi, ulu oya ukuluha ubebe,
   nuulu ukazenga numba yawiza nuulu yibadi yawiza, ehe, bukutuula ha
   budoshi … 'Akulala he? Ulala umu ung'wenuyu'… Hamo utiiko, aliki hamo
   utabatulaga, nuulu hamo utabitaga kinehe, nuulu hamo ukayombelaga
   kinehe? Bakahayaga bo benekili.*

   *Ubudoshi bukenhagwa ulu utuluhaga, busabi. Uyo aluhile atalawilwa
   budoshi … Ung'wene akawilagwa giki baluhi aba. Giko duhu alina ki
   nang'hwe, ung'wenuyu alimulemba duhu kinehe? Al'ubebe ulu uli nasho,
   ulu udomuja kamhayo, aleke, uhaya: 'Mtubonaga, badosa giki'.*

3. *Yaya, ukuyugeniha aliyo ogohaga umu moyo … Baba, nakuwiile, ulu uwilwa
   budoshi, na maisha gako gageehaga. Nuulu giti ikaya yeniyi yuyupandika
   matatizo.* The speaker quoted was the man I cited earlier, who joked that the
   group's envy wouldn't stop him from wearing fancy clothes: 'I will wear
   them all right. But while fearing!'

4. A survey of witches is moreover a recording of names conveyed to the
   interviewer, which tends towards public accusation. Accusation is different
   to suspicion I will argue.

5. Young unrelated women are relative outsiders, hence potentially
   empowering, and allegedly the least prone to a disposition for sorcery. At the
   most they use magical potions for seduction, unless otherwise instructed by
   a witch.

6. *Bandya makanza ga kwila, ku nguno umisa akenhelejiwa giki ubutamu ubo
   twabejiwa nabo, ku nguno ili giki unkima n'ungosha buli munhu ali na
   butamu, butamu wise bo mili. Angu misa mumho bakizunyaga ha kaya.
   Nutenda na ng'hwe, unisagila. Unene natendaga na ng'hwe, hangi nugalucha
   giki gashi unkima uyu heli giki atutosije … Ubeja ishirika lili giki 'Gashi
   umbati ndoshi gete, nalalile na ng'hwe aka!' nkima akategaga.*

7. Ray Abrahams notes that Nyamwezi were already warning about increased
   witchcraft at the moment of migrating into compact settlements in the mid
   1970s (Abrahams 1994: 13).

8. *Ubiise aho twashoka umu kijiji, twazenga sawa. Twahayukituulwa aho tulija
   umu kijiji, twiyogohile gete abanhu. Tutali ikisukuma gete luulu uko
   twandija. Nuulu giti ahenaha mpaga akukugiisha duhu… Waliho boba wa
   giiki: 'Ulu nuleka ukungiisha, nuwilwa giiki "Wali wambitiila ung'wana
   mbati ukija kunigiisha"'. Basi, twahayukituulwa akabala kenako kushila.
   Kiiza kabugimu luulu: nuulu ulimana na ng'hwe waneka duhu. Huna
   wayukumya niyo? Ikijiji shenishi, angu makoye! Basi, twahayukituulwa ikaya
   ijiise ija kwinga kuunu* [names of villages], *jutananha kabuli duhu pyi. Ja
   banigini abadobado, buli kaya.*

9. The modern value of equality, stimulated since the Enlightenment, has this
   experiential source called bewitchment, I will argue in Chapter 7.

10. This translation is derived as follows: *ng'w*(1) -*i*(2) -*bon*(3) -*eel*(4) -*y*(5) -*i*(1); the one who (1) causes (5) to see (3) oneself (2) persistently (4).

11. Some women told me that they were more liable to this type of impulse. They thought eating the liver of an animal may stimulate it, so the liver should be reserved for men. They prohibited their children from eating liver, so as not to corrupt their affective development.

# Chapter 6
# Divination: A Healing Journey

Chapter 2 introduced us to Seele's patients, such as Sara and Albert longing for an oracle to conclude their therapeutic journey. This chapter will discuss the oracle of a patient who had completed treatment. Mashala[1] began therapy as a patient of Seele's father, Lukundula. As is often the case, the story of his affliction is mostly that of a search for the correct diagnosis through divinations. I followed Mashala's case through to the oracles that were consulted in the final stage of his treatment.

Two kinds of divination are commonly practised in Sukuma villages: the mediumistic type (*ng'hambo*) and the chicken oracle (*buchemba wa ngoko*). In the first type the diviner enters an altered state of consciousness after receiving a twig (of the euphorbia bush) to which the subject's saliva has been transmitted. Diviners commence by shaking a gourd rattle or their winnowing basket containing old coins with the twig lying on top. Their ancestral guide speaks through them, or they recollect a dream received the previous night. Diviners who have started their profession following an affliction caused by an ancestor summoning them to carry on their tradition of divining are highly valued. Other diviners, 'those of the fee' (*wa bu-hemba*), have been trained by an established healer. The most common example of divination employed by a trained diviner is the chicken oracle, and it is mostly men who practise this type. The general outlines of its interpretation have become more or less public knowledge.[2] The chicken oracle is often used to cross-check mediumistic diagnosis (as well as to verify ancestral blessing and protection before commencing initiation rituals, see Chapter 3). Chicken diviners, however, are less solicited than acknowledged mediums, because the latter are supposed to acquire the information in a more direct way from the ancestors.

During the two months that followed my *ihane* initiation I was trained in the art of chicken divination by the elders Ng'wana Chonja and Ng'wana Mawe. From the dozen divinations I witnessed and the three I performed myself, I learned that the main challenge is to think like the witch. To do so, the diviner learns to think like the client, who is after all the one bringing a particular witch into existence. The first person singular by which diviners recite the oracle is the 'I' of the client. From the fact that healers learn to think like the bewitched, one should not conclude that they consider the witch a figment of the client's imagination. It is that the witch can be known through her victim. About the witch's identity the diviner has no clue in the empirical sense – if they did, they would not need to rely on ancestral inspiration, dreams or chicken entrails. Any clue will be of a mediumistic kind, which refers to sensitivity to the social environment, to knowledge about the state of the system, and to the creativity of the artist in tune with the subject's experience. Clients have to recognize their problem in the diviner's witch, or else they take their money back. Because of this client-centred approach, it matters little whether or not we as observers reject the existence of the witch. Our attention shifts from the issue of imaginary accounts to the effects (beneficial or not) on the client's condition.

# The Case of Mashala: A Therapeutic Narrative

When I met him in 1995, Mashala, a sociable man in his late thirties, father to six children and officially married to two wives, was about to complete his traditional treatment. Over the next five years I would become privy to his life and history. He lived in our village until the day he publicly made a witchcraft accusation against a neighbouring family, soon after which he and his family left.

His trouble began in 1991 when his mother's cousin came to visit him on her way across the southern part of Lake Victoria. Soon he heard news that she had been held responsible for the death of her husband, and had subsequently been chased from both her daughter's home and later her son's after the inexplicable death of a grandchild during each stay. Mashala's mother wanted her cousin to stay, so she stayed, doing her share of the household work. Mashala

153

watched with some apprehension as his first wife grew close and somewhat attached to the widow, though the latter was avoided by most other family members. People who don't become emotionally involved are less vulnerable to witchcraft. Mashala's worst fears came true in the second year of her stay. His first wife lost a child, and she had experienced excruciating pain during the birth. Just before this another ordeal had left an indelible impression: the death of Mashala's favourite sister, who lived next door. Mashala could bear it no longer and chased the widow away, saying in public that she was destroying his family. Mashala was sure that no relative of his would greet the widow, and at this point she left for Buzinza. Nothing has been heard of her since.

Mashala could not forget the day his sister became ill. She had come back from weeding the cotton field, and she ate as usual. After serving the men, who had taken their place outside in a circle for dinner, she got dizzy when standing up. Her body started to shiver, resembling malarial fever (*degedege*), and then she fainted. When she opened her eyes, she told Mashala that something was exerting pressure on her heart. Whenever the grip on her chest loosened she felt better. Some suggested taking her to the hospital, but others pointed to the sudden development of this illness, suggesting it was witchcraft. The local healer, Ng'wana Busalu, was sent for. The young woman described her state to the healer, how her chest was hurting and her head too. The healer then prepared some roots he had brought along for treatment, mixing the medicinal powder with water, but as he brought the concoction to the patient she fainted again, desperately gasping for air. They decided to wait until she opened her eyes. She never did. It was late at night and pitch-dark. Silence abounded. Outside, all present saw a *chenge* approaching, a bush-fire which appears out of the dark and is associated with witchcraft. It died out on its way to the fence of the homestead.

Puzzled, the family members waited until sunrise to decide what to do next. Some proposed consulting a diviner on the matter in order to establish whether Mashala's sister had really died or whether she had been abducted by witches. Her mother refused, however, and said it would be better to bury her first and finish the mourning period. Those present agreed and that morning at dawn all the neighbours were alerted to the burial. The night following her burial, something remarkable happened. Panic broke out among the mourners in the central yard when they saw the silent shade of the deceased appear. They ran back inside the house, and when they looked outside again the ghost was gone. This happened twice that night. Mashala understood by this that his sister had not died, but had been abducted by a witch. The corpse wrapped in cloth they had buried and smelled was not hers, but a dead animal's placed by the witch or an accomplice.

After two months of deep sadness Mashala decided to go off with his younger brother to figure out what had happened. They travelled to see Lukundula. There, twice in succession a chicken was killed and probed for divination, but every time the oracle refused to reveal itself: the 'canoe seat' (*nhebe*), which indicates ancestral guidance through a haemorrhage detected on the chicken's spleen, was lacking. Lukundula gave the clients the name of a pupil of his, a mediumistic diviner skilful enough to break through the witch's defence. At this medium's compound a young man sitting in the company of elders told them to wait for the diviner who would soon be back. Mashala and his brother sat waiting until they heard the metal sound of *njuga* bells shaking in the *iduku*, the healer's round grass hut, signalling that the clients were welcome to enter. The young man who had told them to wait appeared to be the diviner. He asked for the *ng'hambo* twig for divination. Due to doubts about his sister's death, Mashala handed over a fresh branch to the diviner. He knew that this might put the diviner on the wrong track as a deceased subject requires a dry twig, but Mashala was willing to take the chance and count on the mediumistic skills of his host.

In divination the client discloses no information on the identity of the subject; that is, the afflicted person. Although the subject of divination is usually one of the clients present, it could also be a bedridden patient. The diviner has to tell from the oracle whether the subject is a man or a woman, a child or an adult, in search of healing or just good fortune. The diviner whom Mashala consulted started off by revealing that the oracle concerned a woman, and that she was ill with pains in the chest or in the head. What disturbed him was that he could not perceive her soul (*moyo*). 'But why do my ancestors tell me that this person has gone?' the diviner asked. The reason, he continued, was that this person had fallen ill when the sun was setting, and that she had died even before it rose again. Mashala would not accept the oracle and stood up, claiming a refund. His younger brother, who had no experience with divinatory matters, was fascinated and remained inside the hut until the oracle was finished. It turned out that Mashala had perhaps reacted too impulsively by leaving early. The younger brother was told that this woman represented a case of *litunga*, of apparent death. Nobody had seen that it was not really her body but a dog's corpse that had been buried. According to the oracle, Mashala's sister had been abducted by a neighbour who lived south of their compound. The diviner even described the surroundings of the witch's homestead, the cattle, the number of houses and the total number of inhabitants in that compound. This witch was said to have operated together with two other neighbours, and all three of them had acted by order of their leader, who was kin of the victim.

This description corresponded to Mashala's suspicions. Certain tense encounters with his neighbours in the past now acquired new meaning, such as the time his wife was reproached for refusing to lend out a new skirt. Following a request from Mashala and his brother, the diviner said that he might be able to liberate their sister, but at the cost of one cow and 15,000 Tanzanian shillings (about $30), something which they did not possess at the time. The oracle was later confirmed and further specified by a renowned diviner whom Mashala had visited in the eastern Ntuzu region, where the origin of divination is said to lie. The diviner admitted that he did not have the magic to rescue their sister from her occult imprisonment.

In 1993, not long after he had chased away his mother's cousin, the alleged witch, Mashala became severely ill. The night after he had begun to build an extra house and plaited the roof structure which he would thatch the next day, he woke up with fever and burning pains in his chest, which soon extended to the whole upper right part of his body. The diagnosis at the dispensary was pneumonia. Despite the medicine he bought, the pains got worse. For four days in a row he got an injection at the dispensary, but according to him this only resulted in sleepless nights and increasing pain in his chest and right arm, so he lost faith in medical treatment. Moreover, the time he did manage to fall asleep he was 'able to dream'. The recurring dream showed the cause of his illness and the way to treat it. Despite some friends' advice to go for a more thorough examination at the district hospital in Bukumbi, he had made up his mind that the only way to heal would be 'the Sukuma way'.

Observing the bad state Mashala was in, the continuing high fever and numbness in his right arm, his paternal uncle brought him to a healer for diagnosis. The oracle left little or no room for speculation: Mashala's affliction was sent by a witch, and his life was in peril. The ancestral guide spoke through the mediumistic diviner, who recounted that after returning from a trip to his in-laws, Mashala had stepped on magic destined for him. The evil agency rose in the body from his feet up to his stomach and eventually to his chest. But Mashala escaped certain death thanks to his ancestor who helped to block this magic, preventing it from completing its fatal course by reaching his heart, as the witches had planned, and as had happened earlier to his sister. This ancestor, *guku nkulu, isamva lya ku buta*, his 'great-grandfather' on the paternal side, had posted his protective measure at the edge of Mashala's heart. The ancestor expected his descendant to acknowledge him by wearing in his honour the accessories that used to characterize him during his lifetime: *itendele lyaza*, a copper bracelet, *itendele lya bubote*, a twisted bracelet, *nanga gwa shenu*, a walking stick, *shilungu*, a white shell, *lupingu*, a heart-shaped shell. (The list permits clients to check the value of the oracle, because these accessories and the type of sacrifice or libation made at the altars usually follow clan tradition.) However, the diviner afterwards advised his client not to comply with all the ancestor's wishes for the moment. As the saying goes: *Ngalili akapondelwa bulogo*, 'The generous is ensorcelled for his trouble'. In other words, a satisfied ancestor will not be of much help.

Secondly, the oracle showed that Mashala was suffering from an *ndagu* spell of the *ibona* or 'seeing' type. The diviner warned Mashala that black magic was still lying in wait in his compound, and Mashala realized that he could not return home. So his uncle, who had accompanied him and who was a healer too, proposed that Mashala stayed at his place. That evening, when they approached the house, the uncle began the ritual procedure to extract the *ndagu*. Despite further therapy that night, including concoctions and massages to cure his chest and right arm, little or no improvement was made. From morning until evening Mashala stayed with the other patients, participating in their routines of medicine taking and administering skin anointments. But he felt his problem was of another type, and after five days the uncle agreed to let Mashala go to be treated by Lukundula, the most renowned healer of the clan.

For four days Lukundula performed chicken divinations, but every time this was done a truly remarkable thing happened before the eyes of all present: no signs whatsoever as to the origin and nature of the illness were noticeable. The measures taken by the witches to obscure things seemed to be very effective. In the meanwhile Mashala had lost all his strength and could not walk any longer. Based on his dream and former divinations, he had made his own diagnosis. What he needed was a *luhiga* concoction, which is a 'cold' medicine. According to Mashala, the assistants of Lukundula (who was himself absent) were misled when they claimed that the condition of his body showed that it needed a 'hot' type of treatment. Due to a lack of divinatory guidance, in the confusion about the proper treatment one assistant even speculated that the swollen arm suggested *ibaale*, a swelling of the body, which normally starts from the feet up, like bilharzia. This treatment, however, proved as ineffective as the former ones. Only now did the full array of symptoms begin to appear as predicted and in all their might. When Lukundula finally came back from his trip, the circumstances were right for a major divination to conclude the diagnosis. Lukundula discovered that the *ndagu* Mashala was suffering from belonged to a variant called *mana*: the 'you will know' (*ku-mana*) curse. Consequently, he performed the ritual of expulsion discussed in Chapter 9.

During the following two months Mashala's condition stabilized, but the swelling of his arm had not stopped; it was three times its normal size. From a distance of six inches you could feel the heat his right arm extended. In the meantime, Lukundula's daughter, Seele, gradually improved her mediumistic skills by controlling her spirits. Mashala became very attached to her regular divination sessions, which to him were particularly significant in helping explain his illness and anticipating its future course. Whenever he felt weak, he could draw strength from her oracles, which like his recurrent dreams clearly showed the evil agents in action. In May 1994 the swelling retreated as far as the shoulder, becoming a boil that finally burst. After this Mashala regained his strength and felt cured, and wanted to return home. Yet, only divination could determine whether the danger was really over. Lukundula told his patient that he had not yet seen his 'path' well, so he could not give his formal consent and let him go.

In 1995 Mashala returned to live with his family but paid regular visits to Lukundula. Two years later he had a chicken divined in my company, for he wanted an update on his general condition. The diviner was Ng'wana Chonja, assisted by his friend Ng'wana Mawe, who himself heads the divinations and rituals of initiation in the society of elders. The session took place during the period when these two elders were teaching me the basics of chicken divination. The following account of Mashala's oracle at the same time summarizes what they taught me. I do not possess the ethnographic materials that would enable me to situate their divinatory knowledge historically and cross-culturally. Of the twenty or so divinations sessions I witnessed outside the training context, a handful were chicken oracles. But from numerous conversations on these matters and from accounts of historically significant divinations, I conclude that the tradition transmitted by Ng'wana Chonja and Ng'wana Mawe is largely the one applied by other Sukuma diviners and elders as well.

## Stomach, Gourd and Blessing

Any chicken is fine for divination as long as the subject (who need not be present) has transmitted some saliva to the beak and muttered some words requesting the ancestors to clarify their problem. When the diviner sees a client approaching with a bird in a *kasanzo*, a little cage of branches resembling the ancestral altar, he (it is rare for women to perform chicken divination; they are mostly spirit mediums) makes room on the ground between his feet and lays out a bundle of dried *maswa*, long grass used for roof thatching. He dips the bird's feet, head and wings in a bowl of water for purification (*nzubuka*), hoping to ensure that the oracle overcomes the witch's magic of camouflage. After inserting a reddish grain of sand into the bird's beak, whose solidity is compared to the ancestor, a wet knife caresses the feathers of the wings, while the following words implore:

> You, chicken, show the canoe seat. Travel and come back. You, decoy, collect it all, do not hide anything from us. Tie left hand to right hand. Go from the east, from the great mediumistic healers over there, up to the west.[3]

The bird is placed with its back on the dried grass, both legs spread out, invoking the image of patients confined to their bed. The diviner clenches the left foot with his own right foot and the bird's other foot with his left foot, performing the manual operations of divination in a closed circuit as it were, his body mirroring the chicken's. The diviner identifies with the bird, which itself represents the patient. While the feathers of the left wing are spread open, he swiftly cuts between the joints of the right wing and lets the blood out. In this way the bird does not struggle. The skin is cut from the knees upwards to the neck. Then the right breast is cut loose and the breastbone is pushed to the left to expose the entrails, and the parts that are irrelevant for the oracle – namely the lungs, oesophagus and the crop – are removed. Any traces of blood are washed away with water. The procedure permits a quick methodical overlook. The chicken diviner does not enter a state of trance but adopts a mode of incantation, giving voice to the voyage his exploring fingers undertake in the bowels of the patient's life history.

The first thing that is sought is the ancestor's presence. That is the 'canoe seat' (*nhebe*) referred to in his opening incantation. Diviners are alerted by haemorrhages on the organs. The *nhebe* must be detected near the bird's spleen. It serves as a check on the value of the oracle. Another term for it is 'eye' (*liso*). Without the 'canoe seat', the diviner will throw the dissected bird away and say: 'It has no eyes' (*Iti na miso*). Without the 'canoe seat' there is no divinatory journey because the ancestor has not revealed itself. Ancestral guidance is usually compared to the traditional stool with the broad, encompassing seat. The stool supports the descendant until death, when the stool is split in two and thrown into the grave. Twice I proposed to Paulo that we would dissect a chicken together just to do some review exercises on its entrails before our teachers resumed our training sessions. Paulo laughed my proposal away. The 'canoe seat' would be missing if we were not seeking to clarify some inner state or problem, he said. I checked and coincidentally he happened to be right on those two occasions. There I was, as he said, divining 'nothing but a dead chicken'. Divination is a journey into the unknown, yet securely backed by *nhebe* (*n-tebe*), the 'canoe seat'. As in the *ihane* ritual, the ancestor carries the descendants paddling their way on the river of life. The left hand and the right hand are respectively the subject's patrilateral and matrilateral ancestors.

During divination the diviner holds a lively monologue of successive questions and answers, expressing his relief or anger at what he perceives, as if he were himself the victim. Before the client is expected to reply, the diviner addresses him with a provisional summary of his findings. Here are three fragments from Mashala's oracle. The first one establishes his general state of well-being:

> [Fragment 1]: You chicken, your blessing is fine. But as I began to check your feet, I got angry. When I saw the right foot, I cursed the pains and the illness that began at your ankles ... You, chicken, have I eaten poison? At the mouth it denied so. My poison, I have trodden upon it on foot. When stepping on this, I call it a witch's trap ... The [poison] does not date from yesterday; I got it some time ago. Then my body grew weak and cold. I shivered like a mad person (*mayabu*). The coldness began when the sun arrived at that point. That is what the chick came to tell. However I am fine in the body, except for some muscle aches.[4]

Before engaging in more specified indications of inflicting agencies, the diviner verifies a series of general indicators of health that associate life with containment and tension. Three modes of well-being are distinguished. First of all, to measure the subject's physical strength, the diviner held the bird's duodenal loop, which in oracular speech is called *lubango*, literally 'blessing'. Since it stood erect, the diviner concluded that the subject (whom he did not know yet to be the client, Mashala himself) is not bedridden. That is the meaning of the first sentence in the fragment above. Secondly, the gall bladder (*ndulu*) or 'gourd' (*kisabo*) was full, showing that the subject's body has the capacity to contain. Otherwise the gallbladder will look flat, long and empty. The reasoning here is that digesting food indicates vitality. The combination of a straight *lubango* with an empty *kisabo* points to the danger of heart problems (or some other imperceptible illness). The 'blessing' measures physical strength at the level of muscles and limbs. The 'gourd' attests to the body's internal balance.

The third modus of the individual's well-being is the 'home' (*kaya*) itself, detected on the bird's gizzard or 'stomach' (*ng'humbi*). The association between stomach and home does not refer to the geographical circumscription of the compound, nor to the household as such, but to social status (*lukumo*); that is, to the extended body of supportive social and ancestral affiliations. It stands for social capital in the broadest sense, including the protective medicine enveloping household members. If the gizzard is not fat and swollen but emaciated or pierced then the subject of divination has passed away or is about to; the patient is dead, at least socially, no longer participating in the home's expansion. The body has become a broken shell, like the potsherd symbolising death. More than gourd and blessing, the oracle's stomach is decisive. To observe the 'home' unpierced reassures the patient.

# The Four Dimensions of the Homestead

Next to the stomach, three more dimensions of the homestead structure the oracle. For the sake of analysis they could be termed homes 'of the flesh' (compound), 'of the bone' (household) and 'of the skin' (the ancestral dimension of the homestead). Firstly, a triangular area of flesh on the inside of the right knee depicts the compound as a plot (*ha ng'waalida*). Traces of previous attacks appear there, the vagueness of the haemorrhages determining the time-span. A series of points outside the triangle suggest enemies 'kicking the dew' (*kukomya lume*), setting off before dawn. Secondly, the hip joint (*lukunu*) between the back and the leg denotes the household as a whole. If this bony ball is immaculately white and round, then it is said to reflect the shining teeth of a happy, laughing family. Otherwise the intentions of the witch are made clear: 'Only war on that family'. On the lower back or loin (*nkimbili*) lumbar pains are checked. As usual in Sukuma divination, this one-to-one analogy between chicken and the human anatomy is paralleled by a metaphoric level of association: since the *nkimbili* is situated exactly on the backside of the hipbone, it also represents the head of the household. It connects the leg to the back, motion to life bearing, husband to wife. Any red spot there may considerably coarsen the tone of the oracle, as it reports 'the turning over of the headrest' (*kuhigula* or *kuminula nsago*). The household head has been put in mortal danger by someone for whom he forms the headrest at night, namely by one of his wives. The same suspicion is expressed in the oracular expression *kujuula ikingi*, 'the uprooting of the king' (like a tree). The plan to overthrow the household head should be visible on the white sinew, *kaluge*, on the outer wingbone, where the flight feathers are joined together. A stained *kaluge* marks the interference in the sinewy bond between ego and the protective forefathers.

A fourth dimension of the home concerns the demands of the ancestor, revealed on the chicken's rectum when turned inside out (also symbolising the black garment of the healer). This interior skin, an area representing the ancestral seat, maps out the compound with greyish or other coloured patches resembling the required altars (*magabilo*) and bracelets (*matendele*), which should honour the ancestors in sacrificial rites and therapy. The size of a swelling in this area reveals the intensity of the ancestor's anger. There, at the groin, are also rooted the bird's two long retractor muscles, which divinatory tradition calls *luge*, signifying the tendon of the forearm. Their elasticity measures masculine power and potency, for these muscles between the hand and the elbow allow man to bend his bow (*buta*), the symbol of fatherhood and the patriclan. This masculine power fades when the subject has engaged in extra-marital affairs that were not accompanied by gifts. A black stripe across one of the yellow testes (in the case of a male chick), or on the ovaries (if a female), reveals fertility problems. A next step in the analysis is to check the *luge*, which denotes the client's genitals, *madobelo*. A tainted *luge* signals a venereal disease or an ailment of which the symptoms have a genital nature such as *kisambale*, bilharzia. Any such danger in the area of the *madobelo*, which should be visible on the retractor muscles, can be related to adultery or so-called sexual 'loans' (for which people use the Swahili term *mikopo*) that have not been settled with the lover. It is common understanding among Sukuma that men should in some way pay for casual sex. The reprisal of a mistress, using her lover's sperm in aggressive magic with the help of a female elderly witch, is considered to be of a more innocent kind of witchcraft than that originating from reproach by kin or marital partners. In the oracle the *luge* is male. The spleen, known as 'cooking stone' (*ihiga*), is female. An ulcer on both signifies that if the subject is male, his wife has bewitched him.

Experienced diviners can speculate on the client's therapeutic journey by unravelling the scars located in the 'beds of the past' (*bulili wa kale*) underneath the hipbone, at the base of the *luge*. Of course, in spite of this set of analogies, the oracle remains an interpretative construction. It can head in different directions depending on the moment and on minute signals from the client. For instance, at the base of the *luge* the diviner might not read a 'bed of the past', but opt for a well-known alternative: the paternal aunt also resides there, in the vicinity of the buttocks, at the root of the tendon that symbolizes a man's potency. Like the ancestors, the paternal aunt contributed to the cattle from which her brother drew his offspring.

In the recited fragment the diviner appears to have figured out rapidly that Mashala himself was the subject of divination, who had inserted his saliva into the oracle. This he could make out from the position of the 'canoe seat' (*nhebe*), the subject's protective ancestor. The *nhebe* lay on the left, hence male, side of the chicken's spleen. Had it been on the right side, the subject would have been female. (The client at the same time gets an indication of the oracle's value.) Furthermore, no red marks being visible in the chicken's throat or trachea meant that Mashala had not swallowed poison. Several vague reddish marks could be found on the tip of ribs, on the skinned shoulders and the lower back, suggesting muscle aches and weakness of the patient dating back some time. A split 'tongue' (on the pancreas) would have signified that the patient is the victim of malicious gossip. The pit-like area, where the duodenum takes off from the 'home' (gizzard) heading to the 'tongue' is known as 'in mourning' (*mu nyombe*) or 'grave' (*shigila*). There the diviner's fingers may touch upon a mark resembling a gravestone, which tells him of recent deaths at the client's home. This mark was not found in Mashala's chick.

# Ripened Symptoms and Snakes

A general principle in divination is that significant events, otherwise left at the mercy of our hazy memories, 'run blood red' (*ja-laluka*) on the entrails, on the bones or on the flesh under the skin of the chicken. Another verb is frequently used: 'to ripen' (*ku-hya*). The mass of past events has ripened into these critical points for all to see. Because of the obvious analogies with human organs, direct references can be made to symptoms. A red spot on the bird's brain will be the mark of blows inflicted on the head, especially on the *ng'hooni*, the occipital bone called the 'second heart', which is regarded as very sensitive and prone to sorcerous attack. These blows are perhaps not yet felt, or still at the stage of *masalaaji* (*ga ntwe*), 'shimmering discomfort' announcing serious headaches. Sukuma patients are extremely interoceptive, that is, sensitive to internal bodily changes. Confirmation can be found in the oracle's ribs, *lubazu*, which determine the existence or coming of pain. Problems in the chest, related to breathing or to the heart, are examined on the liver of the bird, which during divination is named *shikuba*, 'chest'.[5] A swelling on this so-called 'chest' points to *mbegesho*, constrictions in the region of the heart, usually accompanied with breathing problems. Other defects, like a hole in the liver, evoke the possibility of tuberculosis, heartburn (*chemba moyo*), or other lung- and heart-related ailments, which are nowadays rarely attributed to witchcraft. Finally, two important anomalies on the *shikuba* should be mentioned. If a piece seems to be carved or loose, about to drop off, then the patient is said to be faced with a very malignant *ndagu*, of the *wahule* type: one chip after another – children and other household members – will 'drop off' at home, killed by this kind of black magic which targets the homestead as a whole (see Chapter 2). Colours or stripes in the middle of the *shikuba* refer to a similar *ndagu*, namely *ndagaja*, eliminating one household member after the other, until nobody is left.

For Sukuma healers, death has set in when the person no longer breathes, *myuye* (breath) being the detectable manifestation of the 'life principle', *moyo*, which itself is located in the area of the heart (*ng'holo*) and chest. Any colour change on the heart of the chicken denotes the ancestor's feeling of neglect. If the heart's shape tends towards a *shilungu*, round shell, or towards a *lupingu*, triangular shell, then the voice of the ancestor has been clearly heard. Their descendant should wear this shell on the heart in the same style as the ancestor did in the past, and they should do this as a token of love and respect. Prominent markings on the 'lake' (*nyanza*) exposed by the ribs of the chicken's back tell the diviner that the patient observes traditions that are proper to the people living at Lake Victoria (the patient may be non-Sukuma). There can be markings for, among others, special altars built in the water at the shore, involving a ritual canoe (*lyato lya malindi*, canoe made of soft wood), skins of otters and the sacrifice of a spotless white hen.

Both hands of the diviner further slide probingly over the intestines (*bula*) to check the colour of their contents, which shine through. He has entered the realm of the 'snakes', *nzoka*, where convulsions – the movements of the snake – may be felt. Pain is the movement of one of the snakes. Elders told me that the snakes are the 'life principle', which connects people to their ancestor. It took me some time before accepting that different forms of pain in the body were materializations of ancestral presence. The most common manifestation of ancestral presence is the 'snake in the stomach' (*nzoka mu nda*), felt as a stomach illness. At the point of death it causes the last spasms and leaves the body. The second snake affliction is located in the head ('snake in the head', *nzoka ya mu ntwe*, also *y'ipungu* or *y'ihuji*) and is accompanied with malarial fever. Other snake afflictions include those of the chest (*mu shikuba*), of men (*ya bagosha*: a child's testicles have not descended), of the tongue (*ya lulimi*), of biting (*ja kuluma*: flatulence), filarial lymphangitis (*ja nghanami*), of blocking the womb from conceiving (*ja buhale*), of diarrhoea (*ja kupanza*), and of the kidneys (*ya lufigo*).

If the content of the intestines looks very black and these spots increase in the direction of the gizzard then food may have been mixed with witchcraft (*bulogi wa kulisha*), which may direct suspicions toward the women cooking. The diviner will verify the throat (*milo*), and cut open the gullet, *ya kulisha* (of food), and trachea, *ya minzi* (of water). Finding red marks here confirms that the subject has swallowed black magic, perhaps a poison leaving the patient with a throat ache. If the diagnosis has until then assumed a fairly harmless tone, then just the throat ache will be mentioned.

Mashala did not worry about food poisoning. The diviner declared: 'You chicken, have I eaten poison? At the mouth it denied so'. However, almost from the start of his exploration the diviner had noticed that one of the pair of appendices at the end of the bird's small intestine was swollen and irregular in shape. The appendices represent the subject's feet (*magulu*). Normally the appendices resemble two black feet each ending in a white tip. Irregularity of the 'feet' makes a strong case for the most feared diagnosis: 'snares' (*mitego*). Might Mashala have stepped on a trap prepared for him? The poison of a snare enters by the feet, rising upwards to the chest, the traces of which can be seen in the clogging together of black spots in the intestines starting from the 'feet'. The magical trap does not always manifest itself in the patient's legs swelling. A magical attack rising upwards from the feet may also cause one of the most common afflictions treated by Sukuma healers, namely *mayabu*, the loss of control over speech and behaviour. The oracle suggests that when the problem started 'some time ago' Mashala may have verged on such a state, which we have seen to be both physical and mental (Chapter 2). He felt 'weak and cold' and 'shivered like *mayabu*'. This is often the consequence of snares (*mitego*). Next to strengthening the ancestral bonds, therapy aims at reversing the course of the poison (see Chapter 9).

Going over the long, coiled ileum of the small intestine, the diviner halts at the 'sleeping' (*bulala*), a tiny outgrowth, which Western biology has coined Meckel's diverticulum. If it does not 'sleep' but stick out, then its tip shows the position of the sun, the time of day when harm was contracted and the symptoms of snares, cold sweat and shivers, began. Mashala's oracle displayed a number of scattered black balls stuck in the small intestine (see Fragment 3, below). These are digested residues (*shipolo*) pointing to 'old traces of the witch's attack' (*bushesha w'ikale*). Since the three modes of the 'life principle' (gourd, blessing, home) showed no important flaws, the diviner deduced that the client has been divined and treated before, and that he might have been prompted to consult the present oracle because of the *kwiluka* danger that most patients are aware of, namely that the scattered remnants increasingly spread out in the intestines and eventually interconnect again into the feared elongated black mass of sorcery. The imagery derives its terrifying character from the oft-employed analogy of fast-growing sweet potato plants (*malando*).[6] Expansion and decrease of black remnants in the oracle's intestines indicate whether or not the witchcraft is reacting to the remedy. For patients, divination is often about that: regularly assessing the progress of treatment.

# On the Joint of the Wing: Identifications

After establishing whether affliction is involved, and tracing its symptoms, the patient's biography should be recounted, as well as the current intentions of the witch. For that reason the diviner ventures onto *mapanda*, the 'cattle tracks'. These paths, marked out by the frequent passage of cattle meandering through fields, refer to the subject's habitual pathways and favourite hangouts outside the compound. They are detected in the form of white lines on the flesh of the chicken's breast, where traps lying in wait can also be found. In Mashala's case the diviner declared:

[Fragment 2]: I came to see those cattle tracks, they are all clear. When I followed the chicken, it came to block itself, standing in the shade. Just waiting, it had left the path. As it was hiding itself, I asked it, when checking the 'tongue', if maybe we are insulting each other at home, or perhaps there is a quarrel at home? The chicken denied. The split in the tongue was only a very small, superficial cut. Then I came to hate the old widow. Those from the neighbourhood are accompanying her. You see the bringer of sorcery, who regularly passes by, at home, at our compound? She comes to check and to become acquainted. She has been given [the sorcery].[7]

A group of haemorrhages was seen at a distance from Mashala's path, meaning that the witch and accomplices were standing 'bashfully in the shade' (*bisunda ha mhelo*) and not where the action is. They fear the protection the patient has been given. On the ribs the diviner discerned the accomplices, 'carriers of the vessel' (*bashenha ndeebo*). They are believed to 'really know' the victim, for example kin or acquaintances who have easy access to the house. Since these were vague reddish marks and close to the tip of the ribs, the actual bewitchment took place long ago. On each side of the bird's breast, somewhere in the middle, something like a nipple is imagined. A haemorrhage there would indicate the patient's witch to be no less than the mother herself: *Alipaala ha lubeele*, 'She is slapping herself on the bosom'. This can be corroborated by a red speck on the inside of the knees or lap, the place where the mother keeps her child for washing and feeding. Other suspects may be women who are in a position of having to grant respect to the patient, such as sisters and wives of younger brothers. Because they must kneel to greet the subject, the oracle designates them with a red speck in the middle of the (left) knee, *izwi*. If it slightly deviates from the middle then the oracle might be dealing with more distant kin.

The oracle culminates in divulging the identity of the bewitching actor by scrutinizing the feathers of the wings (*ma-nana*). In Mashala's case the diviner concluded:

[Fragment 3]: The witch's canoe seat is hidden here at the doorway, so she is kin. Where lies the corresponding feather? The subject of the chicken calls her 'small mother' [maternal aunt]. The subject of the chicken has become self-conceited [*ndoshi*]. The bringer is not family, because that would have been very visible at the knee ... Poisonous remainders from long ago are stuck inside. If they join up they can grow again like a potato plant.

They do spread out, but to say I am in trouble again, no way. That has come to a standstill. If it had been a 'seeing' curse, oh man, you'd still be quite burdened ... Those who are waiting in the shade, their talks sound like if they are afraid. If they still had the need, they would be close to the path, checking constantly whether they could do their job ... So, just keep on using the ordinary medicine.[8]

When it comes to diagnosing a problem, the Sukuma divination system follows the direction of life transmission, namely situating the cause of the problem in ascendant lines. The language is individualistic, not only in the use of the first person singular and in the collective interest in the fate of this one individual. Contrary to the everyday definition of the self as a link in the ongoing succession of clan generations, the patient is here portrayed as the end point of a chain resulting in his present fate. Similarly, in mediumistic divination only the outer twigs of the euphorbia fences surrounding compounds can represent the patient.[9] Divination depicts the subject as the culmination of influences from clan and community. It locates the subject on the joint of the bird's wing (*ha bukonelo*), namely on the junction separating the two main categories of flight feathers, the primaries and secondaries. These two series of feathers respectively correspond to clan (*luganda*) and neighbourhood (*buzenganwa*). Each wing numbers eight generations ranging from the patient's parent up to the founder of the clan.[10]

Once the diviner has reached the 'cattle tracks' and the area around the knee and hipbone, he will check and crosscheck if any of the flight feathers bears a little red mark on its umbilicus (detected after scraping away the down feathers). If he finds one, then the identity of the witch can be revealed. The chicken's first primary feather, representing the patient, is situated at the threshold between clan and neighbourhood. Each subsequent primary feather symbolizes the parent of the previous feather. Left and right wing respectively represent the father's clan (*ku buta*, 'from the bow') and mother's clan (*ku ngongo*, 'from the back'). The small feathers or coverts (*machibya*) in between the flight feathers refer to classificatory kin of the adjacent flight feather. The first feather succeeding that of the subject on the patrilateral wing is the father. The next feather, if tainted, incriminates a paternal uncle (*baba ndo*) or paternal aunt (*sengi*). Then follow the primaries of the three ascending generations alternating between respect (*baba*, father) and joking (*guku*, grandfather): *guku, baba nkulu* ('great-father'), *guku nkulu* ('great grandfather'). The next ancestral figure is *mami nkulu*, the great maternal uncle, also named *wa ku buta migongo*, 'of the bow backs'. He is the maternal uncle of ego's grandfather. He has not fathered the fourth primary, but he sums up (I was told) the influence of men who do not belong to the patriclan yet whose role in life transmission has trickled through via their sisters who have become mothers in ego's clan. The sixth primary stands for *baba nkulu ntale*, the 'great grandfather', father of *guku nkulu*. The last two primaries, or the 'first' two ancestors, are the *mizimbile*, the 'grand great-grandfather', and *iso nkulu*, 'your founding clan-father', also denoted as *makuma*, the great collector. All these paternal ancestors are male, but their wives are included in their name. The primaries of the maternal wing commence with the subject, followed by the mother (*mayu*) and her female relatives: *maama* (grandmother), *mayu nkulu* ('great-mother'), *maama nkulu* ('great-grandmother'). From the fifth primary onwards the maternal wing observes the logic of patrilineal descent along the male line of ascendants: *guku* (grandfather), *baba nkulu* ('great-father'), *guku nkulu* ('great grandfather'), and finally *makuma*, the 'great collector' of that clan.

It is significant that the divinatory wings make no absolute division between the negative influence (haemorrhage) of a witch, such as a paternal aunt, and that of a much older ascendant who is an ancestor. I suspect that this is because their effect comes down to the same thing: both witch and angry ancestor eventually stand for a moral power that kills. *Ndagu*, spell, is the Sukuma word. As I have said, divination is 'to check one's *ndagu*'. The subject wants to know whether they got 'the treatment', whether they need to fear moral power.

A red mark on one of the secondary feathers points to a neighbour. Their identity is tentatively determined according to criteria of spatial proximity. For instance, the fifth feather, counting from the subject as point of reference, earmarks the fifth closest homestead as the source of evil. (Never have I known a client to take this as more than a general indication, so it could more easily confirm existing suspicions about a neighbour.) Some diviners make a distinction between two kinds of secondaries: the neighbourhood proper, which is named 'unit' (*shilumo*), and the villages around or 'the landscape' (*mahanga*, or 'second unit', *shilumo sha kabili*). It is interesting to note that the oracular grid reserves less room for distant strangers as the cause of illness. As divination structures experiences that Sukuma otherwise have spontaneously, it confirms the primacy of the aspect 'moral power'. The oracular grid is not fixed but currently primes for certain kinship positions such as the home's mother (as headrest, knee, doorway, feather).

In the third fragment of the invocation, Mashala's diviner verified the feathers. The chicken disclosed a tiny red point on the female side of the 'doorway' (spleen). This prompted the diviner to look at the maternal wing. On a covert along the second primary of that wing a haemorrhage could be discerned, which indicated a classificatory mother (*mayu ndo*). Mashala's mother's cousin, whom he had chased from his compound, belongs to that category. Mashala thus found his private speculations confirmed by an authority. Of all those present I (who knew Mashala's life story) seemed the most surprised.

The oracle does not present a coherent account from the onset. If the provisional diagnosis obtained from the three modes of the life principle, the four dimensions of the homestead, the cattle tracks, and the intestines suggests a non-lethal affliction, then the diviner will further ignore signs of witchcraft. Divination through the use of entrails has a much more public character than the mediumistic type (*ng'hambo*). The clients themselves are given a chance to peek into the oracle and the diviner may hand it over to an assistant or colleague for a second opinion. Although I never observed it, the client could thus inadvertently influence the oracle at crucial stages.

'Are there any accomplices?' I heard Ng'wana Mawe ask Ng'wana Chonja. They checked the two cavities in the wing bone of the primaries. For a fortune-seeking client the two receptacles in the wing bone relate to the prosperity of clan and homestead. But if witchcraft has come to light, then their meaning changes. The first receptacle, called *izunzu* (pounding vessel), had a red mark exposing the person pounding (*bupondi*) the substances. The second receptacle, called *itale* (the place of drying the medicinal plants), exposed the second accomplice. Confirmation was found in a feather of the neighbourhood incriminating the third homestead away from the subject's. The oracle had found the two accomplices detected at the cattle tracks. They had carefully planned the execution by familiarizing themselves first with the victim's household.

171

Other terms for these accomplices describe specific tasks: *nshisha* (the one who makes sorcery arrive), *ushenha ndeebo* (carrier of the vessel), and *uyo wenha buhwahwa*, the one who brought the lies. Rarely are the words *nogi*, witch, or *bulogi*, witchcraft, pronounced during divination. The Sukuma prefer a more subtle terminology, employing metonymic or metaphoric speech, with a strain of euphemism, such as *mbogoshi*, a little bag to carry medicine, *masala*, tricks, *ku-ihebela*, to play on, *ku-iboneela*, to look upon. In this context terms like *igenge* and *salangaata*, which describe a group of people or clique, are immediately associated with witchcraft. As mentioned earlier, patients usually feel isolated and imagine witches to act as a group.

In short, the divinatory system outlines a cosmology of its own, one in which the subject comes across as an individual occupying a pivotal and solitary position facing the worlds of ancestors, clan and community. An experiential approach abandoning the static view of culture will not seek to affirm this cosmology as typical of Sukuma culture, or reject it as 'un-Sukuma'. Divinatory practice is attuned to a particular experience of the participants. The altered conception of the self in the oracle will turn out to form the ideal breeding ground for diviners to generate a diagnosis that could heal by itself.

## Motives and Claims

What is the motive of someone wishing you dead? In the oracle, each mark of witchcraft is said to have 'ripened'. The expression 'to be ripe' (*ku-hya*) also applies to someone who has been fined by the community. In witchcraft those debts concern claims laid to one's life. As I mentioned before, the traditional word for credit is *shili*, which could be translated literally as 'eating thing' (from *ku-lya*, to eat). A creditor entitled to 'eat' the debtor brings acts of sorcery surprisingly close to community sanctions. Facing possible death, the victims may wonder if the affliction is not altogether justified and if they themselves have not given reason for bewitchment or ancestral sanction. These doubts are expressed in their fantasy of the neighbourhood gossiping about them during the day and intruding into their home at night. In the case of Mashala's divination, during the explorative phase the diviner articulated this anxiety accurately: 'I myself, the chicken, have been labelled as self-complacent' (*Unene ng'wenekili, ngoko, ninikagwa lina lya nyadoshi*).

172

Whether the witch has really given up, and has refrained from the desire to finish the job that they have started, can be learned from the *lwala*, the finger, which is the bird's alula, a small bone or thumb sticking out of the wing. A red point on top of that little sharp bone indicates: *Aliluma lwala*, 'She is biting her finger'. The pointing forefinger temporarily withheld and clasped between her teeth signals that she still has bad intentions regarding the victim. To point, *ku-son(el)a*, is a form of bewitching, while its noun, *soni*, signifies shame. A strong relation exists between bewitching and inducing 'shame', the feeling of being reproachable. In a society where adults witness during their lifetime five or more periods of famine affecting the community and where rains are unevenly spread over fairly small areas, this sense of responsibility over the less fortunate should be no surprise. Therefore, diviners also propose another way of reading the 'finger', namely as a begging hand, called *lulandila*, the borrowing spot (from *ku-landa*, to borrow). It assembles the people with requests (of cash nowadays) that ego has turned down.

Those who lack sufficient provisions might talk behind the victim's back: *Wa-doshiwa tushiliwa*, 'S/he is satiated with food'. By invoking the norm of solidarity they occupy the position of the witch. Norms of social exchange and reciprocity can be negotiated and sometimes broken, without further harm. But in the eyes of the bereaved and afflicted the social game and its law has contracted to a rigid Law (with capital letter). The self is split from the surrounding world and considers the possibility of lethal bewitchment by close family. The witch then fulfils the role of executioner of that Law. Divination in its first phase reproduces this specific experience, which was studied in the previous chapter.

A red mark on the chick's knee, associated with women who kneel when greeting, can refer to an outstanding debt called 'the cows of others' (*ngombe ja bangi*). For instance, in-laws may be suspected of using retaliatory magic, because of an unaccomplished bridewealth payment of the groom. Even if the subject has paid bridewealth and knows of no other dues, he can hardly exclude the possibility of being burdened by a 'cow of the maternal uncle' (*ngombe ya mami*) which he would owe to one of his sister's sons. Nobody can be sure about the actual state of his or her social debts and credits, simply because that balance depends on the opaque gaze of the others. Normally this imaginary gaze dissolves in the social exchange and communication with others. But what about those with whom the patient is structurally unable to exchange? When Mashala suspected his maternal aunt (mother's sister) of bewitching him, he was not reproducing beliefs programmed by his culture. The oracle convinced Mashala when referring to the witch's feelings of neglect. During the two years of her stay the maternal aunt had apparently developed a sufficiently intimate bond with Mashala and his household for him to feel deeply uncomfortable after chasing her. Diviners know that the consultation reaches its peak when it manages to articulate the subject's emotional unrest. The diviner spoke of Mashala's selfishness when disclosing the 'granary' (*ifuma*), a vesicular zone hidden underneath the flesh of the chicken's breast. Detecting a red speck there, the subject meets the eye of the witch fixed on his provisions, on his unshared food (or money). As containers are associated with fertility and success, they are also expected to form a source of envy that can only be defused by the gift that transforms the relationship between self and other. Since gifts within the family achieve no transformation, it is indeed within the kin group that the witch most likely exists.

The diviner knows the anxiety that affliction brings along: how the client has been speculating, alone or in the company of close friends, on the 'what', 'why' and 'who' of the ailment or bad luck. The diviner identifies with the patient's belief that 'the witch is in the home' and he shows he knows very well what it implies. If later in therapy a group or the clan are involved it is because patients experience the social as problematic. They experience a 'generalized Other' within, rather than an external particular other, engaging in magical combat. Moral power is weighing on them. In an ingenious manner Sukuma divination attempts to reverse this inclination towards a generalised Other, and produce a healing effect. Before divination, the evil lingers on as an unidentified 'Other'. As the diviner reveals illness to be caused by an identifiable angry ancestor or vicious neighbour, the patient is breaking with the perspective of a sanctioning Law. Moreover, the very fact of being guided by the ancestor during the oracle disproves the isolation imagined. Therefore the ancestor's presence is crucial. In it the Law itself 'speaks' to the victim. The witch loses her intrusive quality, and her moral power vanishes as she becomes separated from that whole of community, ancestors and clan. Clients feel relieved and invigorated at the end of the diviner's session. Healing rituals, we will see, further specialize in this harnessing of moral power. The ritual publicly shows on whose side the ancestor stands.

# The 'Doorway' in the Oracular Paradigm

Divination becomes rather meaningless without a crisis of variable intensity (from doubts to illness) preoccupying the client. The oracle brings home the crisis first, and from that point reconstructs the world. Divination thus seems a play on experiential frames. In a classic text, Lévi-Strauss (1972: 181,198) has compared shamanism to psychoanalysis. A transference between patient and shaman sets the scene for the 'abreaction' in which trauma could be overcome by reliving its causes. The transference consists in the shaman voicing the inexpressible psychic state of the patient. As the intricate chain of significant moments and social ties that had gravitated around Mashala were unfolded in the oracle, so too could he find his mood reconstructed from the hazy contraction of symptoms, pain, doubts and memories. Lévi-Strauss's story of the Zuni boy (ibid.: 172ff) offers another parallel with Sukuma divination. Once the boy accused of sorcery had admitted his guilt, he was surprisingly absolved by his community, invigorated as it was by this validation of their worldview, which had ended their state of uncertainty. By analogy with this community seeking 'the satisfaction of truth, which is infinitely greater and richer than the satisfaction of justice that would have been achieved by his execution' (ibid.: 174), the distressed individual retrieves his poise thanks to the social recognition of his experience and perspective. So it appears that at the beginning of the consultation the diviner does not shake up the participant's understanding of the situation, nor offer 'a more acceptable world for his client' (Peek 1991: 219). Too many deviations from the client's expectations will jeopardize the identification they have started up. If diviners may have given a paranoid (Turner 1975) or neurotic (Lévi-Strauss 1972) impression, it is only because it has served their profession to verge on the state of mind proper to affliction. Before realigning this state, divination must invoke it.

The diviner explores the chicken's digestive tract from 'home', over 'gourd' and 'tongue', to 'snake' and 'feet' to uncover vulnerable spots, raw emotions and the murderous involvement of family and community members that appear on the oracle's flesh and bone: knee, hip bone, lower back, tendon, breast and wings. The 'canoe seat' (*nhebe*), also known as 'eye' (*liso*), aims to see through everyday life's sham and pretence. It is found on the spleen. The 'canoe seat' of a female subject appears on the 'inside' or right side of the spleen (*nhiga*), the men's on its 'outside' or left (from the bird's angle). The spleen itself is also termed 'cooking stone' (*ihiga*). Manipulating the cooking stone like a shutter, the diviners call it the 'doorway' (*lwigi*) of the oracle. Dividing outside and inside, the doorway represents the main hinge of the divinatory grid. In its gendered division, the doorway actually reproduces a major figure of crisis: on the one hand, women correspond to one term (the right side) in the code male/female, but on the other hand, given the female connotation of both doorway and cooking stone, women outdo men in also embodying the medium itself (the spleen) that constitutes the code. With this simultaneity of code and medium, the divinatory grid evokes the experiential structure of intrusion, which healers associate with the bride and the paternal aunt in particular. Women control the inner sphere of the home that men cannot master.

Divination has little interest in the complementarity of male and female, inside and outside, which is celebrated during the *ihane* rituals of initiation. Sukuma divination does not deal with the dreamy side of sorcery, such as the sabbaths of witches and the nightly sounds of hyenas and owls in popular discourse. Instead, it describes a world where one's source of well-being awakens the neighbour's envy, where partners and close kin seem unfathomable and ancestors are quick-tempered. A unity had grown between Mashala, the diviner and the oracle, after going through the ordeal of reliving the antagonisms in the kin group, the motives of the witch, the expectations of others, the betrayal of insiders at home, the powerlessness of the individual, the history of the illness, and the therapeutic journey. On this mutual attunement the oracle's good news could have full impact. The oracle had shown that Mashala's bewitchment had reached a virtual standstill. Only some black traces of sorcery remained visible *ha baala*, in the large intestine, still far from the stomach. *Tumilaga bugota duhu*, 'Just keep on taking your medicine', was the reassuring conclusion of the diviner.

Paternal and maternal ancestors join at the 'collection point' (*nghumanilo*) of the oracle. This crucial concept is again derived from one of the Sukuma language's most common verbal stems: *ku-kuma*, to collect. This point can be traced in the area beneath the doorway, which is known as *ha mikoba*, 'at the drum straps'. The drum straps are an intersection of white, membranous cords formed by the aorta branching off into two arteries, the celiac (to the stomach) and the cranial mesenteric (to the small intestine). About this intersection, one Sukuma diviner stated: 'The whole of your clan ancestors assemble at the drum straps. Those from the bow are there and those from the back. They come there to meet ... All your ancestors convene for you, they watch over you, they are waiting for you'.[11] Any ulcer in the area from the drum straps to the spleen and the stomach is suggestive of an *ndagu* spell. An ancestor has turned against the descendant. The witch has managed to corrupt this spirit in order to have access to the victim's life. Access, we remember, is essential in all magic, good or bad. Access to someone's life is facilitated by indebtedness and the other's moral power. The *ndagu* ulcer materializes it. The position of the ulcer in relation to the *mikoba*, namely along the left or right drum strap, determines whether the corrupted ancestor belongs to the victim's paternal or maternal line of descent. In Mashala's case the diviner refuted the hypothesis of an *ibona* spell because he had not come across any ulcer in the area of the drum straps. When our teachers Ng'wana Chonja and Ng'wana Mawe said 'The ancestors converge in you', they were pointing at the drum straps. These umbilical cords as it were connect the ascendants to their descendants. It was a relief for Mashala to perceive them supporting him, to see and touch them with his fingers.

# Healing through Identification and Contingency

One purpose of this chapter is to demonstrate the proper healing qualities of divination, an activity often reduced to its diagnostic claims. In this section I want to contextualize my argument in relation to the literature. I distinguish the experiential frame of divination from the frames discussed in previous chapters.

The key to divination is contingency. The 'canoe seat' represents contingency, the unknown or 'real' intervening in a symbolic exchange. Think of any type of divination across the world, from geomancy or reading tea leaves in a cup to mediumistic seances and the interpretation of dreams: all these hinge on an uncontrollable external influence before the interpretation starts. To outsiders the throw of oracular objects before interpretation, or the neuronal combination appearing as a dream, may be pure chance. I prefer the concept contingency in its original, etymological meaning. From the Latin *contingere*, 'to arrive', the word suggests that the event occurring has a place from which it arrived (see also the French for 'occurring': *c'est arrivé*). 'Arrival' emphasizes that more enters the event than the symbolic exchange of people communicating. The event is non-symbolic, or what Lacan called 'the real' (Stroeken 2004). Lacan (1973: 53ff) took it for granted that the real stands for 'pure chance', a non-place. He did not argue this, he merely assumed that his readers were enlightened enough to know that there is nothing 'out there'. As an anthropologist and sympathizer with Sukuma cosmology, however, I propose to use contingency in its original meaning, which leaves open the possibility for chance to be animated, directed by an extra-human agency or realm, known cross-culturally as the spirit world. In the West the concept of contingency has been secularized, or better: de-animated. I would not want to commit the same mistake by going in the opposite direction and re-animate (from *animo*, soul) contingency, thus defending a belief in destiny, as in 'nothing is coincidence', 'providence rules', or 'everything follows its fatal course'. The attractive stance of magic, including divination, is precisely that it leaves both options open, rather than advocating one belief and considering opponents as renegades. That is the gist of my argument about using experiential frames to comprehend magic. My Sukuma friends were not committed to one explanatory model. They too had concepts that denote coincidence, but they only applied these in specific contexts. They spoke of 'wind' (*luyaga*) or 'infinity' (*liwelelo*) – the latter referring to an abstract principle of cosmological creation – to account for cases of misfortune that are not caused by witches or ancestors. Examples of these are failed harvests and calamities (when people cry: *Liwelelo!*) as well as certain children's diseases and Western types of sickness that can only be treated in the hospital.[12] These forms of pure chance supplement what I call animated chance.

178

Another key to divination, a necessary but insufficient condition, is identification. I use identification in its double meaning: firstly, client and diviner empathize via the oracular object; secondly, they single out the witch. Much of the contemporary literature on divination has ignored this second aspect or cloaked it in a mist of claims on the indeterminacy of the oracle. The intimation is that if diviners could be held responsible for witch killings or feuds, it is only very indirectly since their answers remain vague. Of course, as students of divination we would rather not be studying conspiracies with violent consequences, thereby condoning these by treating them as cultural practices. But for all our good intentions, it is hard to ignore a simple datum: Sukuma oracles strive to identify causes, possibly a witch. Clients take their money back if nothing determinate emerges. The Sukuma patients in our case studies visited different types of diviners in various, preferably distant, locations to make sure that the oracle is not a product of local rumours interspersed with skilful conjectures. Remember that at the onset the client gives little or no clue as to the reason for consultation. It is up to the diviner to figure out from the oracle (chicken or dream) whether the subject's problem relates to affliction or to the search for good fortune; whether the subject is a man or a woman; what therapeutic biography has preceded this oracle; what the ancestor's favourite attire was.

Given these identifications and the effort to find the truth, should we be outraged over divinatory practices? (In other words, are colleagues right to be relieved if the diviners they work with are more vague than Sukuma diviners?) One answer would be the neutrality principle: the prerogative of the scientist is to describe events as an outsider without having to judge them. Thus ethnographers could study headhunting in the Philippines or work among the mafia. But this seems to me to be something of a cop-out and I cannot be satisfied with that. First of all, as the reader will have gathered by now, I am no longer an outsider. I doubt that anyone living for two years or more in a community could ever remain an outsider. Secondly, and crucial to my argument, I have come to appreciate the larger social and experiential frame of the practice because of this deeper involvement. I learned that to identify a witch is not to seal her fate. The identification itself has therapeutic effects that terminate the urge to react violently.

Whence the therapeutic effect? The client's problem gets a tangible cause. As the impinging Other becomes a concrete other, the Law becomes law again. In terms of experiential frames the subject has escaped intrusion to return to reciprocity and to the feeling of a negotiable law serving people's struggle for power. The client is ready for a new start. This return has been catalysed by a third experiential frame, an expulsive frame stimulated through divination. In serious illness, healing rituals can durably enact this frame of expulsion, which divination initiated. Healing rites organize exorcism and rebirth. Participants 'die' of their former selves when leaving the forest. Smeared with a black concoction of groundnuts, they leave their 'hot' condition behind in the forest.

To better understand how identification can end the sense of intrusion that Seele's patients, for instance, were coping with, we must look at what distinguishes divination from any other social interaction. For this we turn back to the first key, contingency. Only in divination do we encounter reliance on what I have called contingency, the arrival of the 'real' or chance, animated or not. Many of the traits discerned in divination can be found in other social practices: the exchange of symbols, the diviner's rhetorical powers, the unpredictable nature or 'poetics' of divinatory communication, and both the analytical and intuitive-synthetic modes of cognition employed (Peek 1991: 3–5). Turner (1975) contrasted the diviner's analysis with revelation; Devisch (1993) highlighted the revelatory, open-ended poetics, the diviner's 'world-making'; and Werbner (1989) settled for the play between rhetoric and poetics whereby the diviner reaches a 'truth-on-balance'. 'Wisdom divination' therefore seemed an appropriate term for the social skill that the diviner excels in. In my view all these proposals are correct but insufficient since none ultimately captures how divination differs from other practices. In these proposals oracles might be substituted by just any other ritual or by a consultation with elders. What these authors did not fully acknowledge is the mediumistic dimension, which grounds both poetics and rhetoric, in divination, even in the chicken oracle. Why would clients consult a diviner and not an elder if it were wisdom they were after? Some of the most renowned Sukuma mediums are adolescents. One would not immediately associate their young age with wisdom. They come closer to the 'pale fox' in Dogon divination, at night 'randomly' structuring the divinatory grid by picking nuts from the sand (Griaule and Dieterlen 1986). The young medium resembles the Kaguru villager who was administered hallucinogens to go mad and pick the witch among the villagers gathered (Beidelman 1986). Mediums thank their reputation to something else than wisdom. They have the capacity to embody the spirit. What does such embodiment entail? Amidst its rich symbolism and unfolding discourse, the oracle offers something external and raw, given out of the blue. We called it the 'real'. Some speak of it as the spirit.

Not coincidentally, the very thing that differentiates divination from other practices accounts for the healing effected. The arrival of the unknown, which Sukuma concretize in the ancestral spirit, does something to the client's earlier sense of intrusion. It changes the frame. The ancestor evokes the 'world' the client feared – the community's reproach and conspiracy, sabbaths in the victim's home. As the world 'talks' to the client, it loses its unfathomable and invasive features. In hearing the medium convey the message of the ancestor, or seeing the chicken do so, this 'outside within' is expelled to be transformed into a tangible other with which exchange is possible. Witch unnoticeably becomes ancestor. During the solemn incantations of the diviner receiving the wholehearted attention of the client, I witnessed every time how the moral power that originated from crisis was evoked and subsequently expelled. Whereto? The spirit world is a good place for evil to stay.

The experiential shift is profoundly sensory. Mashala had been experiencing the seeing curse of 'the one who persistently makes one see oneself' (*ng'wiboneeji*). Now that the 'eye' (*liso*) of the ancestor was siding with him, he could expel the witch's intrusive look. The ripened, blood-red attacks were made visible, tangible. During the session, participants get engrossed in this expulsive frame, which detects evil agencies and externalizes the causes, after capturing their deepest fears. Picture the best horror movie you ever saw, but this time with yourself on screen and interacting! The literature's focus on symbols and on communicative exchange disregards this sensory-experiential process and thus misses out on the therapeutic effect for participants. Such an approach will at best offer a variant on the popular way of making light of divination and magic, as ways of offering hope for the desperate. True, the creation of hope, of a 'subjunctive' sphere, permits the desperate to take pragmatic action

(Whyte 1997: 18ff, 67ff). But divination also hands the participants metaphors to embody and to make things change on the spot (Devisch 1993: 169ff). What, however, is embodied? How to capture this reality of meanings, as much material as social, and their transformation? My concept of experiential frames seeks to determine in cross-cultural terms what is transformed.

In discussing divination and healing, anthropologists may give the impression of being engaged in characterizing a culture, typically a non-Western culture. Yet, we know divination is not unique to Sukuma. Moreover, divination does not originate from an everyday perspective on the world. Divination and healing externalize the ancestors, which is not a common frame of experience for users of magic who actually 'live' contingency and are 'being with' their environment. In terms of Figure 4.1, the frame of expulsion belongs to the third column: sacrifice. The witch's demand for 'the cattle of her lap' resembled the harsh logic of commodity exchange, the first column. For patients to snap out of this purified reason and get back to the balance in the middle, Sukuma diviners bring in sacrifice.

In the general terms of our gift/sacrifice comparison, divination is an example of sacrifice. It relies on recognition more than reciprocity. The oracle depends on ancestral presence (will the 'canoe seat' be visible?) and on ancestral inspiration (the ripened spots). There is much less gift logic, less communication, less exchange of locutions as in daily conversation. We have seen that what bewitchment comes down to, its cross-culturally recurring frame, is the social law (the 'code' of the gift) ruling without its 'medium' (sacrifice). A sacrificial practice remedies this lack. The sacrifice consists in imploring the ancestors, without certainty of reply. Those sacrificing reassert the significance of the spirits, those volatile and unknowable beings. Sacrifice thus absorbs the rigid truth of moral power incarnated by the witch. In the following chapter I speculate that moral power, which magic and divination dissuade, keeps on circulating when its role is denied and the unknown is banned from everyday life, to be controlled by (or at least placed in the hands of) institutions such as science, government and Catholic, Pentecostal or other denominations.

What is the meaning of divination? What makes divination specific, distinct from any other practice? As in the previous chapters, I situate the meaning of a practice in the participants' frame of experience – a frame that only exists to the extent that it is related to all other frames of experience. An experiential frame is not a biologically evolved cognitive module, locatable in the brain, whose mechanism is independent from other mechanisms. Frames derive their meaning from a dynamic set of possibilities. They attest to the socially constructed dimension of meaning. Meaning exists in the structure of culture and experience, not in causes. The next chapter demonstrates that if one does not distinguish experiential frames across the flow of social interactions, one will mistakenly associate an entire people with witch killings and lump the latter with magic.

The diviner's statements can be radical. They often confirm the subject's worst suspicions, including ideas about kin trading a life for a life. But well-intentioned anthropologists may have been too quick to downplay these identifications (lest they severely discredit diviners). They did not believe in the possibility of something they once were supposed to stand for (but nowadays in a cosmopolitan world avoid, lest they be called essentialists): cultural difference. They did not believe in cultural difference, at least not enough to consider the possibility that Sukuma normally do not experience truth in the absolute terms Westerners take for granted. How could a straightforward identification of the witch, framed within the reality of magic, lead to killing the witch? The proper reaction is to use counter-magic. The magical frame, its witches, spirits and recipes, unsettles certainties. Surely, as I heard more than once, witches are innovative enough to insert their magical camouflage in oracles to incriminate innocent people. Moreover, individuals do not situate magic's truth in personal cognition but in social discourse, ultimately in the always innovatory politico-medical network that is now connected to the rest of the globe. Above all, if a session goes well, divination restores the magical balance of gift and sacrifice, and with it an attitude to life (an experiential frame) aversive to absolute truths. All these factors make the seemingly obvious, the culprit's execution, far from obvious.

The effect of divination on clients' decisions does resemble the indeterminacy defended by my well-intentioned colleagues, but – we have learned – only after shifts between at least three experiential frames have taken place: from moralist intrusion back to magical reciprocity, thanks to oracular expulsion. Divinatory seances cannot be understood apart from their relation to culture, including initiation, marriage rules, alliance, witchcraft and healing. As I argued in Chapter 2, the problem, as much as the diagnosis and the healing, is systemic.

# Notes

1. All names of patients are fictitious. In an earlier paper on divination (Stroeken 2004) I mentioned this case using the name Mayala. When we later met the patient said he preferred the taken name Mashala.

2. Hans Cory, who set out to ethnographically document ritual and initiatory practices in Sukumaland, devotes a small section to haruspicy, or divination through the use of entrails (Cory 1960: 21–26). It offers little basis for comparison with contemporary material on the subject.

3. *Ubebe, ngoko, ugengeleke nhebe. Usimize butumba na bugili. Ubebe, Kasanzo, ukasanzaga iyoose, kutubisila yaya. Ujunduke nkono gwa lumoso na gwa bulyo. Ufumile kiya, ku bamanga bataale, mpaga ng'weli.*

4. *Bebe ngoko, lubango lwako lwa wiza. Aho nayandigija ku magulu gayo niiza nugakolwa. Aho nagusola ukugulu gumo ugwa niila, niiza nugubyeeda gupandika bung'weeku na busaatu gukwandigijaga umu shing'ongwa ... Ubebe ngoko, nene nalya buganga? Ku nomo yulema giiki nduhu. Ubuganga wane nabuliilaga ku magulu. Aho nabubitila ku magulu, niiza nuwitana giti giki mitego ... Buti w'igolo, nakwiijaga utukanza. Shiku jimo mili gwane gukwitaga lonzwelonzwe, gwiita na lunyili. Nahuhunala giti munhu wa mayabu. Niita kalunyili ulu limi lyashika kunu. Yiiza yusomboola cheene. Aliyo ndi mhola umili, aliyo ndina winogwe.*

5. Diviners are well aware of the difference between the liver, *itema*, and the chest. However, the chicken's lungs are impracticable for divination as they disintegrate. The organ of the heart carries messages in relation to treatment. Moreover, signals emitted by the liver are associated with jealous impulse on the part of the subject, information which is irrelevant to the oracle since the first person singular in the diviner's account, namely the subject, is never a witch ...

6. These are classified as *shilandi*. When I asked Paolo about any classification, he said this category of plants and crops was associated with the female task of weeding, because these plants creep or grow low, criss-crossing the ground. Their uncontrollable and covert nature distinguishes them from the conspicuous, vertically growing crops, with which men identify.

7. *Niiza nugabona mapanda aya, gape. Aho naikubiija ingoko iyi, yiiza yichamika, yubanda ku mheelo kwitegeela, yuyileka inzila. Aho yibisabisaga, nuyibuja giiki aho nalole kalimi, nuulu hamo twiduka mu kaya, nuulu twiita kabufitina mu kaya? Yiiza yulema uku ngoko iyi. Kalimi kene kubi kanhyuujanhyuuja kanyaleele. Niiza nunkolwa umunhu uyu achiililwe atina ngosha. Biiza bifaata n'uyu aha, angu bene ba mu nzengo duhu aba. Wabonaga uyu ushenha ndeebo, huyo akiizaga lukulekule, akiizaga mpaga ha kaya, aha ng'waalida gwiise. Wiza wakumila luulu giiki nene namanilile ho. Winhijiwa luulu.*

184

8. *Iyi nhebe yakwe uyu ilipaganija mu lwigi, iyi yiise iyanyandugu. Hu loya lwayo ululi he? Ung'wenekili ngoko aling'witana mayu ndo. Ung'wenekili ngoko wabiiza ndoshi. Uwenha ati ndugu wane, nguno ulu ali ndugu wane nikahiile geete akazwi … Yimiilile bushesha w'ikale mo. Ulu wisungilija hangi wafuluma giti ilando. Walanda, al'ukuhaya giki ndina bulisokeelwa hangi, nduhu. Yimiilile. Ulu ni kaliho kabona, yii baba, utaali na kanigo … Abakwibandiilaga ku mheelo inyalungalunga yabo, giki boogohile. Ulu giki ni bataali na budaki, ni bali haho na nzila, bali yukulola kila hene giki uyo twitaga imilimo yiise.*

9. Incidentally, euphorbia trees branch out densely, recalling a genealogy.

10. In ancient rituals addressing the totality of ancestors at the house's altars, and not particular ones such as is the case nowadays, Sukuma used to refer to eight generations, named and embodied by eight male ancestors.

11. *Ubudugu ubose bokobanikilaga aha mikoba. Ababuta bali ho na bamigongo bali ho. Huna biize bugusanija ahamo … Abaduguyo pyi bakubanikila hali bebe, bakulanghanila bebe, bakulindila.*

12. There would be two types of HIV, with or without witchcraft, the latter being lethal while the former would be curable through new traditional medicine.

# Chapter 7
# The 'Pure' Reason of Witch Killing

A situation arises. Culture explains it in some way (witch construction) and responds (ritual). In systematic violence, such as witch-hunts, we notice something else: the explanation itself (beliefs) causes violent situations to arise. Students of culture should be wary of limiting witchcraft to this alternative. When culture is allowed to be creative and dynamic, there will be shifting states determining the meaning of magic, such as the 'cool' state (*mhola*) of 'being with', contrasted with the 'hot' state, *busebu*, which Sukuma cast in terms of intrusion, indeed the exact opposite of 'being with'. This chapter starts off by showing that just as the paternal aunt may articulate 'heat', so can the birth of twins and the condition called 'dry womb'. It is extremely rare, though, that belief in these explanations of misfortune would cause anybody to hunt down paternal aunts, twins or 'dry womb' children.

## The Heat of 'Dry Womb'

The logic of witch construction can be classified under the purified state at the extreme left of our comparative table of social exchange: gifts without sacrifice (see Figure 4.1). I discuss two cases analogous to witch constructs. The first is an epidemic in the family, which healers may attribute to an affliction known as 'dry womb' and may recount in terms of failed exchange of semen and blood. The second concerns lasting drought, which turns up questions about anomalous cases of fertility such as the birth of twins.

Before the HIV pandemic began to terrorize Tanzania and other parts of Africa in the 1980s, there had been other sexually transmitted infections with lethal consequences. I collected among Sukuma

186

healers a list of such diseases. They gave me their aetiology, symptoms and medicinal treatment. Some of these were always attributed to witchcraft, others only sometimes, and yet others never. HIV seems not to have dramatically altered the Sukuma epistemology of healing, since healers commonly distinguish two types, the Western type *ya hospitali* (of the hospital) and the 'Sukuma' type caused by black magic.[1] The second, magical type would be curable by counter-magic.

Healers had a special category of sexually transmitted disease for cases when sexual partners and their children die without sharing a particular set of symptoms and without witchcraft accounting for these. Its aetiology paralleled the logic of witchcraft in an illuminating manner. The cause of death in these cases was the surviving parent who as a child was born from a 'dry womb', *nda nyumu* (also *ng'humbi nyumu*). This person's mother had not menstruated prior to conception, either because she was too young, or more commonly because conception had come too soon after the previous delivery.

On the one hand, the belief in 'dry womb', developed by female healers, strikes one as supportive of mothers and young girls. On the other hand, its logic resembles that of gifts without sacrifice, gifts lacking the magical cooling state. Before the womb collects semen (I say 'collect' following the idea among female healers that husbands have to 'sow' their wives regularly to 'empower the child', *kunkuja ng'wana*) it should have released menstrual blood, *mininga*. If no red secretion has left before white semen has entered, then the foetus is said to be in a hot condition (*nsebu*). The husband may make the gift of semen, but without his wife's sacrifice their fruit will scorch all those becoming intimate with it, cursing all sexual partners as well as their offspring (who until the age of five are considered inextricably tied to their mother's health). Hence, ominous is a transactional sort of exchange whereby a child is expected in direct return for the semen given. Gifts are exchanges that require a sacrifice. In dry womb the husband's gift of sperm was deadly hot by lack of sacrifice. Another way of putting it, in terms of the witchcraft discourse of Chapter 5, is that the husband had acted like *ndoshi*, as if already 'full' and needing no exchange. By refraining from the cool move proper to reciprocity, he has called death upon his home. The 'gift and sacrifice' thesis allows anthropologists to leave the fixed domain of 'the occult' and decide where else in society we encounter the structure, while delimiting within the so-called occult a large part (namely magic) where the structure does not hold.

Another example of the logic of commodity transaction explaining heat is when rains fail to come and drought scorches the land. Long ago villagers attributed this to the chief's failure of containing his fertility, such as when a drop of his blood touched the ground. A more popular explanation of drought is the birth of twins. Twins (*mabasa*) used to be associated with the chief, and could live at the chief's court (Bösch 1930). Like the chief (and life giving itself) twins never 'die' (*kucha*). Instead it is said that 'the drum has collapsed' (*kuchibuka ngoma*). The burial of the twin's corpse is called a 'throwing' (*kuponya*). Just as with the chief – fertility never dies – the burial is done secretly at night. In interviews in 1996 and the year after, Makuma, the leader of the *Mabasana* initiatory society of twins, presented to me a contemporary version of the role of twins. The parents of twins are 'bursters' (*batanduki*). They collect a plentiful supply (*kukwija*) in return for the man's gift of semen. Why would the birth of twins account for the lack of rains? As I interpret it, the sacrificial side is missing in births that exceed one child. According to Makuma, the consequence of the birth of twins would be either drought in the community or death in the homestead (as in 'dry womb'). Makuma's initiatory association proposes to domesticate this excess of fertility by making up for the missing sacrifice. The sacrificial procedure seeks to restore containment. Containing oneself, one's feelings, is deemed essential for adults. As in the myth of the broken water jar explaining the origin of death, non-containment announces disaster.

First, the *Mabasana* ritual specialist *ngangi* (a neologism derived from the Bantu word for healer, -*ganga*) anoints the hair of the twins with the 'beer of shaving' (*walwa wa bumoga*) and shaves it off with an iron blade. The link with the ceremony of *busunzuula*, the shaving of the chief to announce the rains, is explicit. Then ashes, sand and branches from the house are collected (*kuyabula*) and added to the beer in a small gourd to metonymically relate the twins' house to the society's medicine. The rain medicine proper is a 'cold' recipe, calling up fresh rains (*bugota wa bugingi mbula*). The ritual specialist takes the gourd to a pond and buries it at the bottom. More containment of twin fertility is done after the parents return from the forest where they accomplish a ritual passage reminiscent of *ihane* initiation. In the *Mabasana* initiation I witnessed in 1996 they came out painted black and were chased by their teachers. Finally, during a collective dance they showed the baby twins to the community. The twins were lying in a winnowing basket together with two flacon-shaped gourds (*mafinga*) tied together (like the beer gourd in the *ihane*). The twin gourds were afterwards tied to one of the v-shaped legs at the head side of the parental bed. Makuma specified that the *mafinga* should not touch the ground, for there death resides. After this ritual containment, the twins would no longer 'obstruct the rains' (*balemegije mbula*).

# Cultural Creativity and Blind Belief

Are Sukuma convinced, as if applying a science of their own, that every premature conception of a child will later result in the death of that child's partner and children? Will Sukuma exclaim at the birth of twins: 'So this means no rain this year, guys'? The questions spring from a mechanistic worldview.

Many twin births have never been treated, and the rains did come. Many premature conceptions occurred, and there was no epidemic. Rather than building a science of their own, Sukuma have several experiential frames to perceive the world. They are not unfamiliar with the rigid, legalist and, in itself, rational logic of transaction (gift without sacrifice) whereby an investment proportionally returns. But that mechanistic frame serves to explain crises a posteriori. A Sukuma healer who predicts an epidemic in the family or drought whenever noticing a 'gift without sacrifice', such as a too young mother or a birth of twins, would be no different from scientists applying the laws of nature. It would be nothing short of attributing a rigid cognitive state to Sukuma. It would be as if they applied culture without the mediation of experience. It is only in certain, mostly Western, social circles that the mechanistic logic prevails irrespective of changing experience and that any views deviating from it are religious or artistic. We have seen that the West's socialization thesis in its latest, praxiological, guise fails to elicit the experiential dynamic. To correct praxiology I do not propose to add agency or 'subjectivity' to Bourdieu's cultural structures (cf. Ortner 2006). On the contrary, my proposal is to pin down the structures – which are social because referring to forms of exchange – in subjective

189

experience. For anything to exist for us as humans, the whole of reality (with all its bits and pieces collected from the past) has to pass through some structure. But there are many structures.

This chapter argues that it takes a rigid kind of structure to act systematically on the basis of cultural beliefs. There have been examples of cultures labelling newborns with anomalies (such as premature birth and other traits which medical doctors now know to be harmless) as 'witch children', to be killed on the spot (see Sargent 1989). While this may be sound from a Darwinian perspective, I contend that we are entitled to be deeply disenchanted by the practice. This does not mean, however, that the culture as a whole should be repudiated. Our approach allows us to dismiss the particular frame in it whereby socialized beliefs blindly elicit actions. This chapter goes one step further to revisit the Western popular association of 'traditional' cultures with blind belief, which for a wide audience remains the reason for violence in Africa, including the genocide in Rwanda and Burundi.[2] What if the opposite were true, their modernity being the cause of it? If we define modernity as an experiential structure rather than a historical period, could we not accordingly explain the witch-craze at the brink of European modernity? An anthropological reaction to our compatriots' indignation over violence in the Great Lakes has been to point to our hidden role in that violence, hence to replace the role of culture by economic and political antecedents. Yet, such antecedents, as studied among others by de Heusch (1966; 1995), Vansina (2004) and De Lame (2005), will always have a cultural dimension. The structures or frames I have been deriving are a way to discuss patterns in that dimension.

I have argued that in the Sukuma case the more common frame is another one than that of conviction and mechanistic predictability. I have illustrated the repercussions in several domains of society. Users of magic reproduce a sense of 'being with' their environment. Illustrative of this point is the following conversation. A Sukuma elder shared with Paulo and me his ability to live with danger, with nonlinearity, with the dependence of the giver on the receiver. Men depend on women, who occupy a special mediatory place, one of 'stashing' (*kubinda*) men.

> ELDER: In matters of witchcraft men can come to be involved. But especially women manifest themselves in this, because women

exceed in that they – well, to clarify the issue: the reason is that a woman retains much secretion. Take the example of an adulterous woman who prostitutes herself because she wants to get some cash. And her husband doesn't hate her for it: 'Let her just look for things'. But when you have come to agree with that woman, and after the deed you start dodging her so as to avoid giving that money, well then she may think: 'Say, that guy is very much a *ndoshi*, he wants to avoid me, he plays the fool on me and scorns my husband'. So she will look for me, because women collect us, male children. And you see, mister, women have a clitoris. You know that women have a clitoris; and what it's like? They have a clitoris there underneath, a clitoris which male children like, and from underneath which people are born. So at the time of sleeping with her, she will gather everything the man discharges from the onset of copulation. So they collect us, they stash us.

PAULO: Stashing in what way?

ELDER: Collecting you during intercourse. She is covering it with her buttocks, isn't she? Meaning that everything that is in your body, she collects. There should be *ndagu* (fate), she is collecting as you are inside her. Therefore, when you've finished and she takes out your stuff, she is extracting you. And with that she can do whatever she pleases. So that's the issue, there she gets a grip on you, while we, men, do not have that.

Every act of sexual intercourse potentially kills. If women stash men's bodily fluids to make magical potions and control men, why don't men do something about it? That is not the tenor of the conversation. One lives with contingency.

# Witch Killing

QUESTIONER: What is the worst thing you came up against in your career?

DIVINER: It happened again last week. You remember the young man we pulled off his bicycle? He was completely upset. I had read his divination twig (*ng'hambo*). His mother came up in my dream as the person responsible for his wife's death.

These are the words I remember from a diviner from the village in which I lived. I am not sure what he meant. According to Paulo, he was saying that if we had not stopped the young man he would have gone to slash his mother with a machete. He continued: 'That is how rampant witchcraft has become these days'. I noticed a contradiction between the horrific mistake of killing an innocent mother and the supposed fact of an increasing number of mothers secretly poisoning their children. Both, however, fit within the experiential structure of crisis. Paulo and the diviner were summing up the change I often heard the village was undergoing. This change was not only about new practices after increased contact with the rest of the country through radio, public transport and urban migration. The change happens on a less visible and less discursive plane, that of the frame in which practices and information are experienced. I would argue that while the diversity of cultural inventions increases, the plurality of experiential frames is in jeopardy, and with it the dynamic that dissuades the effect of 'truth' pronounced by the diviner in the instance above. The result of this disciplining of people's experience could very well be a surge of witch killings.

This chapter deals with witch killings, a phenomenon that according to the national and international media plagues the Sukuma people in particular.[3] Simply put, my argument is that the Sukuma way of dealing with a suspected witch is not murder. They commonly resort to counter-magic and ritual to regain ancestral blessing and protection. It takes a lot of despair and perhaps even disbelief in magic to resort to the machete. I disagree that animists treat magic and machetes as interchangeable tools of violence. Magic has a contingent, sacrificial dimension that is absent in the machete and in other tools that give a predictable return for energy invested. The healer's plants are informed with ancestral consent; the witch's attack has it too. Accounts of witch-hunts in Africa throughout the twentieth century confirm my data on the witch killer's profile (Douglas 1970; Willis 1970; Auslander 1993; Yamba 1997; Rutherford 1999): they are often schooled, unmarried young men that have not been socialized into magic, such as via *ihane* initiation.

The collective witch-hunt differs from the witch murder ordered within the family or neighbourhood. The latter has extremely personal and intersubjective traits, explicable from the intrusion frame discussed earlier. Although no less horrific, the witch-hunt looks more like an expulsive practice. The tenor differs. As Schoeneman (1975) shows, especially during the colonial period, witch-hunts in various parts of Africa occurred in the context of a social movement announcing cultural change. Afterwards, witch-hunts got into disrepute in that community. I do not infer from this the necessity of a historicist paradigm-switch, like that of John Parker (2004), who reduces witchcraft and anti-witchcraft to historical processes and denies them a reality as structural beliefs and practices socialized. If we give up the implied homogenous concept of culture, we realize that the (experiential) difference between the secret killing of a suspect and the effervescent witch-hunt after public accusation during a historical transition does not exclude their belonging to the same cosmology, as distinct structures.

As I participated in day-to-day activities in Lukundula's compound and spent more time with patients deemed bewitched, a number of questions came to the fore. Why must the occurrence of death have a reason? Why is death thought to have a personalized agency, commonly called the witch (using black magic)? Why is the witch primarily thought of as kin, an insider, who knows the victim? Why is the victim primarily an ascendant? Why mostly women? Why mostly elderly women? If the witch is kin and an elderly woman, why is she then portrayed in generalized (impersonal) discourse as perverted, operating in the world of the night, thus endowed with the features of an absolute outsider, opposite to the social order? Why the paternal aunt?

Instead of having each practice correspond to a certain 'Sukuma belief', I described an experiential dynamic. Equating culture with a set of beliefs leads to absurdities such as the expectation that the labelling of paternal aunts (*sengi*) as witches will lead to the extermination of all paternal aunts. Such a perspective on culture would resemble the aforementioned reaction to an oracle by the schoolboy pulled off his bike. This very approach, however, underlies the decision of the Tanzanian authorities to prohibit divination, because they assume diviners to be pivotal in witch killings. One would think that their assumption is common sense (and reproach African politicians for their laxity for insufficiently prosecuting diviners). What makes their assumption seem commonsensical is our academically ingrained disregard for the experiential in culture. The same assumption about witchcraft beliefs shines through in the recent silencing of the witch in studies of divination.[4] But common sense can be treacherous. A quick calculation suffices to cast serious doubt on the causal link between oracles and witch killing. If every Sukuma village has one diviner with two customers a day, and if on average half of the oracles identify a witch (which from my observations they do), then about a thousand Sukuma villages would annually yield more than 300,000 identifications of witches. About every day a witch should be killed in each village. Even after subtraction of overlapping identifications, it would mean decimation of the Sukuma population. Common sense has seriously overlooked something. It has overlooked the experiential fact that divination can heal, thus preventing retaliation. That is where the magical balance of gift and sacrifice comes in, how it is breached and restored.

# Persecution and Individualism

In a village neighbouring the one I lived in resided an elderly man with few resources who had obtained a mere handful of cows for the marriage of his only daughter. Before he died he had used them all up, leaving virtually nothing for his children to inherit. In the meantime his oldest son had founded his own homestead. He had cultivated his land well and became prosperous, with a herd of over sixty head of cattle. When his sister wanted to divorce her husband, the latter demanded his bridewealth back. Since the oldest son usually inherits the responsibilities of the father, she requested the cattle from her prosperous brother. However, the brother refused, claiming that her problem was not his since his father had left nothing behind for him. His reasoning went against tradition. His duty relates to the clan to which his wealth contributes, and whose ancestors blessed him. A duty should not be interpreted in terms of debt and credit with his father (see Chapter 3). So the sister brought her brother to court in the district headquarters, and villagers speculated that witchcraft would be used at any moment. Eventually, the brother agreed to pay back his sister's bridewealth, five head of cattle, and a rumour spread that the brother was afraid for the fate of his children. Some thought his sister might be a witch. Soon after this it turned out that she had not in fact divorced her husband but was continuing to live with him and was keeping the returned bridewealth cattle for the sake of her household. The brother did not intervene though. The five head of cattle did not breed well in their poor environment and either died or were sold in a matter of years, and soon after this the sister's husband died. Once this happened she was, however, welcome to move to live at her brother's compound.

Ominous constructs of 'the witch' had no doubt popped up on several occasions on both sides. But now magical balance was restored. Everyone was back to square one: 'Aren't we all witches?'. In this frame the witch is just a user of magic.

Virtually any intense emotion, conflict or unforeseeable event can be related to magic if it coincides with crisis. An unfaithful husband dying of Aids, a girl robbed of her favourite dress, someone stepping into a whirlwind, a disputed royal succession followed by the new chief's death, someone's enemy struck by lightning, a young woman losing her child some time after she had refused to lend out a dress to a neighbour, a bag of medicinal objects in a cave containing a piece of skin allegedly belonging to a murdered witch, a bad harvest surrounded by prosperous fields, a successful businessman with a mentally retarded son, disagreement over the return of goods after divorce, a family suffering from inexplicably decreased food supplies, a pregnant woman fearing the envy of her childless neighbour: these form only a fraction of the cases my assistants and I collected. But the moral power called the witch is not sustained for long.

The situation I observed almost daily at Lukundula's and later Seele's compound was clients going home visibly relieved after divination, ready for a new beginning. A witch exposed by the oracle was greeted in person the next morning if they happened to meet. Clients retrieved their capacity to have opposite worlds coexist, such as that of ancestral truth and general uncertainty, of the living and the dead. They retrieved the capacity for inclusive disjunctiveness (the very capacity that obstructs clear-cut ethnography). It is ironic that some anthropologists insist we do justice to people's 'strong belief' in witchcraft (Ashforth 2000, 2001: 220). Nothing could be more modern than the belief in truths leading to systematic action (see 'believed belief'; Stroeken 2008a). Bond and Ciekawy (2001: 6) write in the same vein: 'Whether witches do or do not exist is unimportant; the relevant issue is that people believe they do'. Or as the well-known pragmatist variant goes, witchcraft is real because it is real in its consequences. In other words, witchcraft beliefs predict actions just as scientific knowledge does, the only difference being the tragic fictitiousness of the former. I have argued instead that the relevant issue in deciding on meaning is not people's belief, but the distinct and varying frames in which people (from any culture) experience their beliefs. So the issue for the anthropologist is not to respect another culture's irrational belief, but to consider that culture's variety of experiential frames. As the formula in Figure 4.2 illustrated, meaning (m) includes experience (e). The disjunctive frame of magic keeps options open. This disjunctive capacity disappears among those clinging to truths inculcated by Church, Catholic, Pentecostal or other, by media or governmental institutions. Far from being relieved about the increasing number of young Sukuma conforming to these various institutions' aversion to diviners and healing cults, I am concerned about what happens to the witch in a frame that takes beliefs literally. One indication is the sudden violence against so-called witch-children in south-east Nigeria where the Liberty Gospel Church attracts a large following among people avidly watching its films on witch-children and reading its books detailing measures of detection, in striking resemblance to the 'Hammer of Witches' in 1486 by Kramer and Sprenger, Inquisitors of the Catholic Church.[5]

Early in my fieldwork it struck me that those Tanzanians who seemed obsessed with witchcraft and suffered from it were members of Christian educated elites who publicly denounced its existence and treatments. If one cannot go to a diviner nor participate in an expulsive rite, what does one do? 'The witch' endures. What then does one do? I got to know some members of the political elite pretty well over the years. A middle-aged Sukuma, K– lived in the small town that was the district's headquarters. Amongst colleagues he had the reputation of being an intelligent and charming superior, who did not stand on authority and loved to gossip freely with his subordinates. This image of diurnal joviality was combined with a nocturnal one of lust. His ambitions to run for office in the national elections were no secret, nor were his numerous escapades with local barmaids. This conspicuous promiscuity made some think that the chief's court, where he had grown up, had been an inspiration. I could not help picturing him as an adept user of magic. But one day he confided his fears to me, telling me about inexplicable noises at night and doors flying open. His friend, and colleague, was bothered by similar events. Every night he heard someone whispering at his window. The terror was visibly wearing him out. Both K– and his colleague usually spent the evening in bars and returned home late in the town's only car. K– wondered aloud if the inexplicable events had anything to do with the former inhabitants of the place where they lived. These people had been chased away by the government so that the offices and compounds where he and his colleague lived and worked could be built. It seemed like he was accusing himself. Both lived isolated at the edge of town together with mostly non-Sukuma, away from any community that could show signs of disapproval. And yet, there they were, feeling haunted. K– and his colleague were not feared as witches by anyone around, but they apparently had every reason to fear bewitchment themselves.

Statistics about witch killings in the regions of Mwanza and Shinyanga, where most Sukuma live, have regularly made the headlines in Tanzanian newspapers. In 2002, the news channel BBC World devoted two pieces to the efforts of internationally sponsored non-governmental development projects to combat witchcraft beliefs in Sukuma villages. The news served to illustrate a stream of reports on witch killings in Africa and Asia, and so-called *muti* murders (the mutilation of innocent victims to use their body parts in magical recipes) in Southern Africa. The Sukuma had the dubious honour of figuring centrally in a statistical study by economist Miguel (2005) on poverty and witch killing, a paper much cited in that field. Miguel detected a correlation in Sukuma villages (in Meatu district) between witch-killing rates and periods of drought, which led him to picture the hair-raising scenario of household heads deciding to eliminate unproductive elderly women. Finally, Isak Niehaus's (2001a) seminal book on contemporary South Africa at focal moments cites the 'Sakuma' (*sic*) as an extreme example of witchcraft beliefs turning violent because of poverty and inadequate government policy.

A Tanzanian scholar, Simeon Mesaki, conducted a baseline survey in the late 1990s for the Sukumaland Old Women's Programme (SOWP) in Magu district, sponsored by HelpAge International. The title of this online document, 'Gendercide in Rural Tanzania: Sukuma Witch Killings', is as evocative as that of a report he cites: 'Tanzania's Silent Holocaust'.[6] No doubt, the new NGOs internationally sponsored to combat the killing of elderly women in Tanzania appreciate the logic of an occult form of genocide taking place just to the east of Rwanda and Burundi. Mesaki (1994) had earlier made his name by presenting figures about witch killings, which will not leave the staunchest relativist unmoved. Is refraining from judgment about witchcraft beliefs not to condone the killing of innocent people? Recent essays by Green (2005) and by Green and Mesaki (2005) call for social engagement, warning anthropologists about analytical discourse that itself further institutionalizes witchcraft. Green and Mesaki recount the violence 'in the northwest [of Tanzania], notably among the Sukuma, the country's largest ethnic group' and make the contrast with more 'benign' witch cleansing in the south (ibid.: 374). The authors typify witch killings as 'northwestern Tanzanian (Sukuma) responses' (ibid.: 382). The brackets probably only make it worse for the reputation of this group of 5 million Africans.

Is it not a continuation of the colonial project to replace magic by more 'benign' beliefs through schooling, science and Christianity? On returning from Tanzania in 1997 I wondered what had sparked off this feeding frenzy in the media, both popular and academic. The reports characterized the divination procedures of longstanding tradition, which I had meticulously studied, as ludicrous guessing games by charlatans recklessly inciting their clients to violence. Had I been blinded by my academic interest, or was I kept in the dark when the killings took place? Black magic was a regular theme of conversation. And I had lived in villages so had firsthand knowledge. But from 1995 until 1997 – the supposed peak of the witch-hunts – I had heard of only one person killed after being identified as witch. She was a poor widow living on her own – no burden on any household for that matter. Very often the witches are elderly widows living at the periphery of the village, cultivating their little fields – hardly in keeping with Miguel's (2005) scenario of calculated murder to spare food supplies. For myself, I never doubted the murdered woman's innocence. A relative of hers had attributed the death of his two children to the grudge she supposedly held for being deserted by her family. This man could not find peace and hired a reputed killer, who cut the witch's body up into parts. Why into parts? The body dismembered, existing in bits-and-pieces: this is how psychoanalysts describe psychotic views of the body (see Grosz 1990). Does this not point to an act of extreme emotion, to exorcize the witch's haunting presence for good? Might the killer realize in the act that the significance of the feared moral power far exceeds that of the concrete individual attacked, and hence will not disappear by simply ending that person's life? An abstraction is harder to kill.[7] In any case, we could not be further away from Miguel's (2005) scenario of rational choice, the workings of *Homo economicus*. Rather, we are much closer to the dark domain of moral power such as guilt feelings about the peripheral position of an elderly woman. Economists do not talk about this domain. It has also been conspicuously amiss in the by now large body of literature on contemporary witchcraft in Africa. Clearly, we should not associate the domain of moral power with the Sukuma people alone and presume to have discovered something problematic about witchcraft beliefs as such.

Much of the outrage about witchcraft beliefs and divination is based on a mistaken concept of culture, which lacks the experiential dynamic I observed in Seele's compound. It is time we investigate the statistics that are supposed to support this negative image of Sukuma people (and that reproduce the mistaken concept of culture). One question immediately springs to mind. Would the number of 389 killings over 10 years in a province of South Africa sound as 'alarming' had their motive not been locally categorized as 'witchcraft-related' (Niehaus 2001b: 184)? The word witchcraft in itself has a mystifying effect on Westerners. Sukuma use the word in less charged fashion. That is why I opted for the word 'moral power' to translate their many references to witchcraft such as *ndagu* (fate, curse), *shili* (debt, 'eating thing'), *ibona* (the vengeful look), *ng'wiboneeji* (the witch, 'the one making one see oneself persistently') and the claim of 'the cattle of my lap', *ng'ombe ja matango gane*.

Not only is witchcraft a mystifying term. Sukuma themselves tend to be mystified by their compatriots. In Hyden's term, these inhabitants of Mwanza and Shinyanga region form 'an uncaptured peasantry' (Hyden 1980). They are publicly perceived as such since the failed centralization of their villages. This image of them did not improve when they subsequently created village vigilantes, Sungusungu, to provide the safety and social security the government could not (see Abrahams 1987). It is in this context that one should read the headlines in Tanzania's leading national newspaper about 318 elderly people reported killed in Mwanza region between 1993 and 1998.[8] But what does the figure of 64 witch killings per year actually mean on a population of 2.5 million? Anthropologists have to undertake cultural comparison, or it will be left to quantitative researchers to decide.

The question is especially relevant if witchcraft is used as a local term to report violent death. Furthermore, the registering police officers, mostly non-Sukuma, are known to use the category lightly. Associating Sukuma with the occult is a denial of shared human experience (as well as a dissociation of their culture from recognizable experiences), something which civil servants stationed in Sukuma villages may engage in to justify their unabated corruption but which social scientists should be the last to condone.[9] Seasoned ethnographers, such as Brandström (1990), have always reversed the question: How do Sukuma and Nyamwezi manage to cope with injustice by national authorities and keep the peace in their semi-arid, densely populated land, while welcoming immigrants?

The witch is always an insider; killing her is a crime of passion. Homicides among relatives or acquaintances exist in the West too. In fact, that is the most common situation in which people are killed (more than armed robbery). For example, in a Western region of comparable population density (and with sufficiently detailed statistics), the state of California in the US, the annual rate for this category of homicides is 5.28 per 100,0000 inhabitants.[10] For all the outrage about Sukuma, this figure is more than double the rate of 2.52 witch killings reported in Mwanza region. A silent Holocaust? Anyone objecting that the Sukuma cases might be underreported should contemplate one statistic, kept by every village council: the total homicide rate. As Miguel (2005: 1160) remarks, albeit in a footnote, the total homicide rate in Sukuma villages is below that in the West. We must conclude that international outrage boils down to the fact that the homicides occurring in Sukuma villages do not exhibit the Western age and gender division – for example, there are comparatively more young male victims in the U.S. and Europe. In short, the outrage is ethnocentric. What ruined the Sukuma reputation is, above all, their common use of a word whose translation, 'witch', mesmerizes moderns.

Ethnographic research is an account of culture that draws on an ethnographer's experiences, which themselves are culturally determined, thus raising the question of the researcher's cultural bias. Green and Mesaki (2005: 374) do not ask this question when they contrast 'violent Sukuma' responses with 'more benign' practices and they illustrate these with the phenomenon of witch cleansing in southern Tanzania, whereby a healer in town shaves the body of both witch and victim. Benign indeed, but hardly comparable. The killings are not a cultural phenomenon like the ritual of cleansing. On the contrary, they are a tragic response to the fact of protective magic, divination and healing rites failing to work as endurably as they used to. I have argued in Chapter 4 that the reason imputed to the witch, of trading a life for a life, is a rigid logic, purified of Sukuma tradition.

Life is commoditized – reduced to social law. The victim who responds by resorting to the machete is perfectly in line with this logic. The killer of the witch acts out of pure reason. Sacrifice and witch killing may appear alike, both being forms of ritual violence, but once we include their experiential frames the practices turn out to have very different meanings. Killing a witch is not Sukuma culture at work. The media reports and the academics speaking of the Sukuma response took this for granted.

One more element is indicative of the fact that witch killing does not emanate from the experiential dynamic of magic we have described until now. Killing may reduce the anxiety of the bewitched for a while, but it cannot change anything fundamentally since it does not break with the frame of intrusion; rather, it continues it. The *ndagu*, one's cursed fate, is not dealt with. The moral power arising from crisis lingers on after the witch's death.

When is murder, as an alternative to ritual, most likely? Ritual fails to work if the experiential frame of intrusion is institutionalized, as it is by Church and State. Then the healing experiential shift that ends intrusion cannot take place. More development and less belief in the power of magic, which outsiders see as the solution to the problem they perceive to beset Sukuma farmers, will only further hamper the shift. I am not arguing that Green and Mesaki have reasoned incorrectly. But as anthropologists they should have defended the other view as well. As I discussed in Chapter 1, much of the literature today gives the impression that witchcraft beliefs and practices are symptoms of a postcolonial society torn by poverty and the effects of neoliberalism. People would be at a loss about the new social inequalities they face under modernity. One might almost forget that the magical practices that count as symptoms of disruption predate colonization. What, then, are those Africanists who argue this view implying about precolonial Africa? Is their certitude about the unacceptability of these beliefs the reason for their advocating a discourse that sees only 'modernities' in contemporary Africa? Anthropologists used to gain respect for treating traditional concepts such as witchcraft in a different way. Not that we should respect traditions purely on principle. But we should not forget that traditions may have originated from, and survived, long-term collective trial and errors. Rationalists are known first and foremost to respect what their individual reason tells them to. Yet, traditions may have a collective reason with experiential benefits which elude our individual reason. Pursuing this idea further, we might have to go so far as to argue the same about traditions that, to our individual reason, seem unsustainable, such as the culturally legitimated public witch-hunt (which I would not equate with the private witch killings I have discussed up to now) and variants such as excommunication. How can we be certain that their effect – such as collective well-being at the expense of the unlucky few – is not what would have prevented twentieth-century Europe and the U.S. from cultivating aggression through world wars and global economic exploitation? A similar example is the dubious certainty by which some development anthropologists in Tanzania call 'poor' what many Sukuma consider a lifestyle. Students of culture should not universalize their individual reason.

This brings us back to the role of diviners in witch killings. As my analysis in terms of experiential frames has demonstrated, oracles cannot be compared to court verdicts or to consultations with wise elders. Divination is a ritual with therapeutic effects for participants. Prohibiting divination will more likely increase witch killings. During several visits outside Mwanza region between 1995 and 1997 my assistants and I observed a smaller presence of diviners in villages in Shinyanga region, where divination is forbidden by regional ordinance. Resultingly, if one accepts the idea that divination leads to witch killings, one would expect a smaller number of witch killings here in comparison to our region. Going by figures from the local newspaper, a total of 325 so-called witches were killed in Shinyanga region over three years,[11] which makes an annual number of over 100, more than in Mwanza region, and this in a smaller population. As I mentioned, statistics on these issues are unreliable (with over- or underreporting both in Shinyanga and Mwanza), but they do not seem to support the purported common sense view of district authorities and cited anthropologists alike. My thesis about the role of experiential frames expects an expulsive and soothing effect to come from divination in terms of the client's attitude to life. By prohibiting divination, a sense endures of matters being left unattended and the afflicted miss the divinatory easing of tension. The two years of initiatory healing which Seele offers to her patients cannot be replaced by a quick cleansing rite. Moderns, as attested to by the local development projects I worked with, wish that Sukuma relied on hard data in their attributions of responsibility for witchcraft. On closer inspection, and painfully ironically, exactly this emphasis on a modern concept of truth could set off violence on a systematic scale for it would turn oracular practices into solid bases for action. It would undermine the purpose of magic initiation, to accept contingency rather than combat contingency. Mildly put, it is risky to intervene in people's framing of experience. It is advisable to let a culture spontaneously design new practices in adaptation to their changed environment. I know this will not yet shake the confidence of the many among us who believe wholeheartedly in the progress claimed by the metropolitan wealthy and educated the world over. Therefore, the next section proposes to considerably up the ante and touch on a traumatizing instance of violence, one possibly latently preoccupying the reader: the genocide that has left a scar on Africa's public image, possibly as deep as the Holocaust on European history.

# The Ever Modern and the Execution of the Other

Would the world be better off from banning magic? If it is any indication, the relatively high levels of Christianization and of school education in Rwanda and Burundi did not prevent the genocide in 1994. Longman demonstrates that 'the culpability of the churches lies not only in their historic role in teaching obedience to state authority and in constructing ethnic identities but also in their modern role as centers of social, political, and economic power, allied with the state, actively practicing ethnic discrimination, and working to preserve the status quo' (Longman 2001: 140). In the same volume, de Lespinay writes that a 'significant part of the literature published after the Rwanda genocide by both Catholic and Protestant clergy and concerning Rwanda, Burundi, and the eastern regions of the former Zaire shows clearly that men of the church have been continuously involved in manipulating consciences before, during, and after the genocide' (de Lespinay 2001: 169). About churches he adds, 'how dangerous they remain (until proven otherwise) for populations which, to this day, are culturally alien to them' (ibid.: 169). The 'culture' underlying institutional religion (and perhaps positivist science) is alien in contracting the world into one experiential frame. The genocide of almost a million people in three months raises the question how the opposition between Tutsi and Hutu identity could have been abused by political leaders despite it being a construct (through local negotiations as well as Belgian colonization, cf. Heusch 1995; Malkki 1995). How come the blame works, and this in a society that seemed to have collectively 'liberated' itself from the healing rites and magic that preoccupies many Sukuma? I would argue that the liberation meant substitution of one worldview by a more stringent one. How could someone be convinced of the evil intentions of a category of people such as the paternal aunt, or the Tutsi? Besides the many contingent historical and political factors playing a role, the above suggests a pattern or structure at work: the disciplining of experience. Are social scientists able today to consider the hypothesis that the genocide operated on the basis of belief in an absolute truth (about the other) deemed to be valid across space and time, hence having the potential to quickly cross village boundaries and circumvent traditional intuitions of uncertainty, persuading an unbounded mass of people, which resulted in systematic violence? In my view an experiential structure proper to the situation, and in that sense applicable to humans as such, has more explanatory force and is less essentialist than a structure characterizing the local culture (cf. Taylor 1999).

The level of schooling and Christianization in Rwanda was high in comparison to neighbouring areas.[12] The Sukuma healers I worked with daily did not seem to realize that, since colonization, magical practice has had such a bad reputation among educated Africans and Europeans that associating a people with it has come to be seen as denigrating. Indeed, no matter what the literature may tell us about the many modernities that make up postcolonial Africa, it seems that one frame dominates modernities, stimulated by Church, school, government and civil society, namely the quest for 'development'. The quest says there are truths out there, written, decontextualized, that one can believe in and base actions on. I cannot forget the strong conviction of a Seventh-Day Adventist in Misungwi who pulled me into his living room to accept the word of God and to promise to him that I would stay away from the village where I was working. I cannot help but think of Mashala and Albert in the village, who in the privacy of their room defended to me their fixed, 'believed' belief and summed up the evidence about their personal witch, her motives and past attacks. The rigidity of logic was part of their bewitchment. Rituals of sacrifice in the village might restore the magical balance and its flexible (disjunctive) epistemology. But for the alternative structure to persist without violence, a change of epistemology and an incessant effort of empirical verification would be required, as in the West.

Disenchanted individuals distrust traditional enchantments. They search for 'truth', something arising not from the past or the future but 'now'. They turn against themselves, critical of thoughts entering their mind, always open to the possibility that these may be idols inculcated by culture. In the modern frame, only the 'now' counts, the recent, after the etymological (Italian) stem *modo*, 'recently', in the term 'modernity'. Think of Descartes scrutinizing his thoughts. After thus externalizing the mind, he pictured matter as external to the mind – hence the dualism of mind and body. He placed himself in a position of existential self-doubt, distrusting everything that did not come from within the self. He was left with 'clear and distinct ideas' – hence rationalism. The modern frame of experience is to purify reason from its ties to culture (Gellner 1992). This search for pure reason is not limited to a historical epoch or a place. Postmodernism, cultural relativism and our own discipline's crisis of representation continue this focus on the recent and its mistrust of the idols of tradition.

I claim to have come across modernity in the quaternary table covering ritual practices (see Figure 4.1). When Sukuma patients disenchanted their world to detect the cause of evil, we discovered moments of the 'ever modern'. In viscerally suspecting, for example, the paternal aunt, she who claims the 'cattle of her lap', they rejected the traditional distinction between gift and sacrifice. They put their trust in purified reason, only taking the commodity logic of the witch seriously. The witch construct arises from existential doubt about the world and about oneself in the face of crisis. Patients shared with me their 'clear and distinct idea' when they divulged to me the one they suspected of a secret death wish. Latour's (1993) provocative thesis might as well be inverted: we have always been modern – sometimes. Descartes in Seele's compound: that could be Albert or Mashala at moments when they distinctively pictured their witch to me. Remember the lady on Albert's picture staring straight into the camera lens. Had he taken his machete and paid her a visit, then the newspapers would have said that Sukuma culture got the better of him. I would have to keep quiet, knowing but unable to prove that it was precisely his rationalism that persisted.

Systematic violence is not the only outcome of the intrusion frame. Much less horrific things can come out of it. In fact, some of the norms and values we are most proud of stem from that frame. The challenge is not to abolish this frame but to leave it as part of a wider experiential palette. Western cultures did not invent this frame, their 'modern' society only invented ways to sustain it. By calling the frame 'ever modern' we don't reduce it to a certain space or time. The frames we talk of are holistic realities, properties of meaning-making, rather than mechanistic causalities perceivable in matter or mind. Once we accept this limitation of our analysis, we can push the comparison a step further. What does it mean for a Sukuma farmer, man or woman, to claim that women have made a sacrifice to support the gift system of clans? It is to be critical of the traditional view. It is to reject the value of relating gift and sacrifice, which Sukuma norms and initiatory practices reproduce. The bewitched transcend the distinction between gift and sacrifice and obtain a clear and distinct idea. Their ruminating about the 'cattle of the bride's lap' basically says that society has ill-treated women by keeping them outside the gift system. This idea, originating from a condition of crisis, in fact recalls the Western concept of gender equality. Stronger still, it resembles the position of Western feminists. Grosz captures well Irigaray's emphatic contrast between the multivocality of femininity and masculinity's 'singular meanings, hierarchical organization, polar oppositions, subject/predicate division, intertranslatability of concepts' (Grosz 1990: 180), which preserve women's oppression, while in fact 'social order covers over the debt culture owes to maternity. The son cannot accept the debt of life, body, nourishment' (ibid.: 181) and thus he resorts to 'God, theory, culture to disavow this foundational, unspeakable debt' (ibid.). Sukuma initiation reassures men and women that the social order is such that there is no debt of life raging savagely. It is thus that the idea of an irremediable debt can at all express the breach of social order for the Sukuma bewitched. In this light, Western modernity can be portrayed as stimulating the experiential frame of bewitchment against the magical balance. Moderns have learned to enjoy and sustain the intrusion that generates the values they cherish. Is crisis not the ultimate state of scientists, obsessively pointing the gun of criticism at themselves? For our European values, such as gender equality and empiricism, which became stronger from 1650 to 1750 in the aftermath of our own witch-hunts (cf. Israel 2001: vi), we may have this experiential structure to thank. I called it purification in our table of social exchange (Figure 4.1). The table aspired to non-essentialism by differentiating experiences without reserving these for one or the other culture. So the value of gender equality could fit under the intrusive structure. It undermines the claim the West might have of having invented this value. An experiential frame, not limited to any culture but proper to meaning-making, accounts for gender equality. The moral power claimed by feminists is part of that frame, and potentially violent, but fertile if well harnessed.

## The State, Modernity and Violence

The reader may have been unsettled by the link between Sukuma witch killings and the genocide in Rwanda and Burundi. Might there be anything more to this than the similarity of the seeming irrationality of the violence, the excess, the machete? Rwanda, Burundi and Sukumaland lie fairly near to one another, situated around the interlacustrine Great Lakes region of east Central Africa. In the minds of Sukuma farmers, kings have come from this region, known as *ng'weli* (the west) – for example, the Bulima king claims to descend from a Ha dynasty from Kigoma. In return for obedience, kings would guarantee the rains, the fertility of the land, and would work together with a council of villagers housed at the royal court. Their family members intermarried with the local Bantu groups. However, my evidence for comparing witch killings to the genocide is not historical. It is analytical, with all its due limitations. It considers the systematic violence of both. Comparing the experiential frame of moral power, truth and commodity logic to the experiential frame of magic, gift and sacrifice, it suggests that the historical replacement of magical practice by institutions of truth may result in a reduction in means to deal with crisis, and hence a sustaining of the sense of crisis. The switch from cultural description to social process is common in anthropology. A famous example is the extended case method developed by Gluckman's Manchester school (see Evens and Handelman 2006). Since the 1980s, however, our discipline went through a crisis of representation which questioned the author's right and capacity of representing another culture in writing (Fabian 1983; Clifford 1988; Pels and Nencel 1991). While realizing that our ethnographies were largely a product of our (academic) culture, we kept on writing about 'witchcraft', 'ritual', 'initiation', 'conflict', 'power' and so on, as if our concepts had no culture of their own. How to escape these what I call 'tacit sociologies' and their alternative, the extremely modest (ultra-Geertzian) position offering mere description? My option has been to analyze local practices through a cultural comparison, and to always make the switch explicit from description to analysis.

Siegel similarly makes the connection between witch killings and state-organized genocide in Java. He writes largely in agreement with a number of studies of European witch hunts: 'Instead of a village figure from whom one could demand restitution for harm suffered, the witch now seen by jurists and theologians was in league with the devil' (Siegel 2006: 18). The shift from a concrete person to a figure shattering the social order and menacing the State led to systematic hunts for witches. He earlier observed that in Evans-Pritchard's days witch killings were rare in Zande society. Sukuma elders told me the same. In modern African states the situation seems different. Siegel's reasoning can be schematized as differentiating village and State in terms of their type of witch as well as their way of dealing with witches.

---

Village: Witch (I) = concrete other     $\rightarrow$ (a) restitution (common) or

                                           (b) witch killing (rare)

State: Witch (II) = abstract Other (devil) $\rightarrow$ (b) witch killing (common)

Figure 7.1: Village and State witch killings

---

Siegel's analysis is attractive as it confirms what many ethnographers observe today: violence, including witch-hunts, increases with modern state formation. Another merit of Siegel's analysis is that he rejects the stereotypical association between witch killings and village life. My query, however, lies with Siegel's historical reading of the difference between village and State. His reference to the devil and to the State's violent reaction to presumed hidden threats implicitly opposes two types of culture, each corresponding to a distinct frame of experience, which the reader should recognize by now. The villager's witch can be concretely named and accused for using magic against people (witch type I). The modern State's witch would be an unfathomable Other with capital 'O' (witch type II). Because this abstract witch prevents restitution, such as through the divinatory and healing rituals I have described, the logical consequence would be more violence. Siegel's analysis agrees with mine, except for one crucial point. Where my data from healer compounds disagree is in the idea that the second type of witch (seemingly advanced because more abstract) would not emerge in the village. I have elaborately demonstrated the shift between frames available to humans. How come Siegel does not see the experiential shifts? The idea of a historical evolution from type I to type II is almost inevitable in tacit sociologies that unnoticeably switch between their data on a particular culture and their assumption of a social process (e.g., modernization). That is the price of an historical analysis that sacrifices the experiential factor and with it the search for the meaning of Sukuma witches in Western terms, which might have revealed unforeseen commonalities. The concrete named witch (type I) can be found in Sukuma villages, in public discourse and divination, but it is preceded by a less readily conveyed abstract figure of crisis. The latter figure has all the traits of the unfathomable Other, the type II witch obsessing State officials (whether in Java or Tanzania). This intrusive agent, an absolute outsider within, the antithesis of reciprocity, is the primary witch that healers deal with. It is in no way a second, evolved type, as Siegel suggests. It is the original witch, emerging at the birth of crisis. Moderns in the West know this unfathomable cause of crisis well from their own experience, but Sukuma healing rituals have been better at dealing with it.

I am not arguing that moderns believe in the devil, but that moderns are used to not making evil concrete (which is virtually the same) and that they will attempt to exterminate this abstract cause. For instance, we attribute 9/11 to a religion, nation or social process. No matter how discursively complex our theories may be, their underlying structure of experience has not moved away from the original state of crisis, a rigid commodity logic that humans and groups cling to in crisis. The pure reason of the witch continues to reign for those refusing to shift to an experiential structure of reciprocity with the unknown and contingent, such as the spirits in the Sukuma network.

# Culpability: The Witchcraft within Modernity

The question of modernity and witchcraft beliefs refers back to a research tradition in West Africa on the prophet Atcho and his community of followers in Ivory Coast. In a volume dedicated to the topic, Augé and Zempléni follow Ortigues and Ortigues (1966) in conceiving of persecution (including witchcraft beliefs) as a cultural model and as a stage in an evolutionary process. Interiorization of culpability, whereby patients confess their guilt (as in the prophet's Church) would constitute a break with the persecution beliefs of traditional societies. It would be a next step in the process towards individualization characteristic of modern society (Augé 1975: 230ff). As should be clear from my analysis, I do not consider the model of persecution as a societal stage preceding the interiorization of culpability, for the simple reason that interiorized culpability is the condition for the model of persecution. Ritualized persecution is therapeutic. It is a fairly ingenious cultural construct in response to the Other (or Law) emerging for all humans in crisis. The alleged habit of accused Azande to denounce their double as the source of evil (with a phrase like 'I did not know to have witchcraft evil in me, but if so, please excuse me') is as much interiorized culpability as it is a discourse of persecution. I thus approximate Zempléni's stance on diabolic confessions in prophetic churches being therapeutic for curbing the subject's interiorization of guilt (Zempléni 1975: 213). Zempléni disagreed with Augé's sociological analysis according to which prophetism is a tribunal blocking the patients' consciousness of class oppression. Both authors however associated traditional societies with the model of persecution. Both accentuated the *logique lignagère* ('lineage logic') in village life, people's submission to the elders (ibid.: 215). They contrasted this logic with the competition and self-assertion of the urban context. Individualization would be a socio-historical shift from lineage logic to its counterpart. Yet, is there no individual competition in the village outside the clan? Both authors reason in terms of social process and cultural ideal-type, rather than frames, so they conclude on historical shifts. I propose experiential shifts instead. Beliefs in witchcraft can change or disappear, but the experience of bewitchment – if defined in the subdued terms of a structure holistically related to all other human experiences – is of all times.

Further support for my analysis, and for the holistic quality (cross-cultural validity) of the frames proposed, may be found in Macfarlane (1999: 164, 174, 196), who noted that European witches were often associated with the intrusive presence of a moralist figure, incarnating traditional rules of solidarity that obstructed the rise of modernity. Belief in witchcraft died down in Europe, but not the experiential structure of bewitchment. Yet, sacrifice was discarded and with it the expulsion of bewitchment. The frame of bewitchment took on new guises. A hypothesis worthy of historical investigation may be whether the purified transactional calculus of the witch's reason turned out beneficial in the field of science and technology. One could not have foretold this from its rootedness in existential questions about illness, misfortune and death. One could have, though, when considering the immense creativity of magical remedies aroused by the pure reason cultivated in the healer's compound. My Sukuma friends, at least, agreed that the healer's inventions evoke the Western technological inventions they often marvelled at.

More confirmation of the witchcraft in modernity can be found in modernity's formative years from the early nineteenth century until the mid twentieth century, when a sense of intrusion came to rule inspiration in art and literature. I am thinking of the Gothic wave of *Frankenstein*, *Dr Jekyll and Mr Hyde* and *Dracula* ('This evil rooted within all good'), the critiques of capitalism since Marx and of modernization cited earlier, and the later dystopias of Huxley and Orwell. Had Latour (1993) taken his own culture as seriously as any other culture, he would have realized that the modern search for a purity of reason that isolated something 'natural' – that is, something unpolluted by culture – had cross-cultural relevance and went hand in hand with the deep sense of 'intrusion' that he repeatedly noted about modern Western thought. Does psychoanalytic theory, which posits the existence of a monstrous agency within, not experientially remind one of witch constructs? As I have suggested before, does Habermas's colonization thesis not do so too? Surely, this must shed a very different light on the anthropologist's contention that witchcraft beliefs have to be combated through poverty relief programmes because Africans with greater material security 'would be less concerned about other people being able to afflict them through witchcraft.... [C]oncerns about witchcraft might even come to be subsumed under categories of individual "psychological" disturbance' (Ashforth 2001: 221). Do these psychological theories not attract Westerners for the same reason as witch constructs are attractive to Sukuma patients: they articulate an experience of intrusion. Why, then, would beliefs in magic be the problem, and not the frame of certainty be the source of violence?

# Notes

1. See also the discussion of *mayabu* in Chapter 2.
2. Attributing the genocide to capitalist pressures these African cultures could not deal with is a variant argument (see Chapter 1).
3. The truth of this assertion can be validated by entering 'Sukuma' into the search engine facility of such websites as that of the BBC, Al-Jazeera and YouTube. Since 2008 there have been many reports about another form of witchcraft-related violence presumably popular in lakeside towns among fishermen and artisanal miners looking for a lucky catch: the killing of people suffering with albinism, to use their shiny skin and bones as ingredients for magic to obtain *mwanga*, 'light', namely a fish in the lake or a gold nugget in the pit. Note that such bland one-to-one analogies (suggesting nothing less than the discovery of a natural law) were not the object of magic initiation in our village cult.
4. I thank Wouter Van Beek, co-organizer of a two-day conference in Leiden on African divination, for puzzling over why my contribution was the only one mentioning witch identification in oracles.
5. See the BBC documentary by Joost Van Der Valk et al., 'Saving Africa's witch children', which won the 2009 BAFTA award (Current affairs). Note however the documentary's problematic assumption that witchcraft beliefs mean the same for everyone, hence that Pentecostal pastors continue the work of traditional healers. I again refer to our discussion of Figure 4.2.
6. Mesaki's document, "Gendercide in Rural Tanzania: Sukuma Witch-killings", is listed at: http://www.gendercide.org/links.html. I myself retrieved the document from: http://www.ifra-nairobi.net/new/crime%20 conference %20 papers/mesaki.pdf, retrieved 19 March 2007.
7. After the hit man's arrest in 1998, my informants in the district noted a drop in killings.
8. See *Daily News*, 11 March 1999.
9. I have never seen police officers show up in the village where I worked. (Do they not feel at ease? Do they think the sight of a uniform there looks ludicrous?) To make an arrest they send young men who are in military training. This happened in 1998 to a diviner I worked with. Soon after

Mashala's wife lost her baby, Mashala had accused a neighbouring couple in his new village of trying to drive him away in order to procure the nice house he had built. The public accusation is grave, but sometimes the start of an exchange. However, accusations of witchcraft are against Tanzanian law. The couple chose to use this alternative interpretation offered by the State. They brought charges against Mashala at the police office in town. The diviner was arrested for inciting violence through divination. However, the police were not interested in pursuing the case through the official channels of justice. The diviner was released after paying a bribe, a large sum of money worth three head of cattle.

10. The Californian figure becomes 7.22 if the same proportion is applied to the unknown cases. Source: "Homicide Crimes by Relationship of Victim to Offender", retrieved 19 March 2007 from: http://caag.state.ca.us/cjsc/publications/homicide/hm02/Dtabs.pdf.

11. See *Mzalendo*, 4 October 1998.

12. It may be worthwhile contemplating the extremely small number of Rwandans – 0.1 per cent – who claim today to embrace 'traditional indigenous beliefs'. This needs setting beside the following figures for religious identification: 56.5 per cent Roman Catholic; 26 per cent Protestant, 11.1 per cent Seventh-Day Adventist; 4.6 per cent Muslim; 1.7 per cent claim no religious affiliation. Source: United States Bureau of Democracy, Human Rights and Labour. 2007. 'International Religious Freedom Report 2007: Rwanda'. Retrieved 14 September 2007 from: http://www.state.gov/g/drl/rls/irf/2007/90115.htm. I doubt one would find that percentage of traditional belief even in Europe. Although a fraction may be only nominally Christian, their answer seems indicative of the social undesirability of magic.

# Chapter 8
# Spirit Possession: Incarnating Moral Power

When all therapeutic means, including hospital medication and ritual sacrifice, have been exhausted and yet failed to alleviate the patient's condition, diviners may claim that the oracles have been misread. The source of affliction is deemed not to be caused by witchcraft or ancestral grudge, nor the pure chance of 'infinity' or 'wind' of illnesses hospital doctors can treat. The fever, pain or loss of control are symptoms of an ancestral call that remains to be understood. It is assumed that the person's ancestral guide was a healer in his or her own lifetime and now wants the tradition to be continued. This means initiation into a healing cult.

Bantu-speaking Africa has a long tradition of healing cults (see, e.g., Janzen 1992; Devisch 1993), of which spirit possession cults form a special category. The latter accommodate the participant's mediumistic potential, which initially manifests itself as spirit possession. In what follows we will discuss the *Chwezi* (or *Chweeji*) spirit cult, which is of particular relevance to the topic of moral power. It offers a radical alternative to the witchcraft idiom by claiming that intrusions are the workings of spirits. The cult will help the inflicted to feel at ease with their spirit. The initiated learn to cherish the spirit and whatever intense desire or indignation accompanies possession.[1] Moral power is not expelled, nor harnessed and passed on to burden the next in line. Rather, it is given a stage for all to see. After the witch's stare and the diviner's probing eye, the sense of vision here gets another tenor yet again. Going back to the discussion of divination (see Chapter 6), mediumship freezes as it were the transition from intrusion to expulsion, namely the moment when the diviner and the spirit (or oracle) are one. It is the moment when social redress has not yet occurred, while moral power surges in the form of pointing fingers and ripened ulcers. I propose looking at the spirit's presence in the possessed medium as an incarnation of moral power.

The *Chwezi* cult, I argue, is less concerned with social redress than with the articulation of feelings such as misgivings about the situation of women and their sacrifice as brides. In the *Chwezi* songs we can make out what the possessed's screams are about. They lament, for instance, the bride's unfair exclusion from the gift system. Whilst the gender equality of the cult reverses the common division of male and female worlds, we are not dealing with Victor Turner's (1967) anti-structure in the liminal phase of ritual – that is, announcing social redress after wedding the traditional norm to a positive emotion. The technical aspects of ritual should not blind us to the fact that *Chwezi* men and women consider their equality as the appropriate relationship in the cult (a person's spirit is what counts, and it may be male or female) and that on returning to their daily, indeed gendered, tasks at home they still value the cult's norms highly. Cultural change happens here before the ethnographer's eyes, but what has prevented it from being detected is the Western concept of cultural change. Western sociologists picture a dialectic in which gender equality is a foreign concept in a culture unless it has durably affected the local tradition of gender roles. The assumption is of one experiential frame governing a culture. Change would consist in rejection of one view, substitution by its antithesis, followed by a synthesis. However, in a society where experiential frames are permitted to exist next and in conjunction with each other, people can be radically transformed – enraptured for life by the spirit – while being able to return to their daily life without deserting traditional norms. This experiential freedom, nonlinearity and plurality undermining linear change has hampered conversion to new creeds, religious or political, which has been a source of frustration for *ujamaa* leaders, including Tanzania's founding president Julius Nyerere.

It is important to note in this respect that the redress of social order obtained through divination and healing can hardly be deemed a return to hegemonic order. Following Victor Turner, Jean Comaroff (1985) suggested this about precolonial initiation rites in contrast with Charismatic churches in South Africa. We have seen on the contrary that the purpose of initiation and healing, which is to

215

become a user of magic, amounts to (re)gaining disjunctive freedom after a static state. To apply Don Handelman's (1998) theory of ritual, it would be more accurate to state that spirit possession and Charismatic seances mirror the participant's condition, and by extension the state of the system, whereas healing rites and initiation transform the participant's condition in function of society's desired model. Only, the Sukuma model, I would add, outplays the theory by stimulating disjunctive freedom and plurality of experiential structures.

Another reason why spirit possession should very much concern students of witchcraft (who, as I hope to have demonstrated by now, are also students of moral power) is the strong resemblance between the loss of control among patients condemned by a dead relative to continue a tradition and the loss of control among *mayabu* patients cursed by a living relative: one patient is possessed by a spirit, the other is 'possessed' by a witch. Remember the first column in Figure 4.1: the witch possesses her victim, for she 'owns' him; or, actively put, the victim 'owes' the witch. It is on the basis of commodity logic that she has moral power over him. The passive version, being possessed, is the logic of the fourth column: pure sacrifice, signalling not a shred of self-concern. Spirit possession could be one Sukuma practice that belongs to this fourth frame. Between those two extremes lay the magical balance, the philosophy of 'being with'. The first and fourth column we dubbed 'modern' purifications – for example, money versus friendship, desire versus love. The table's holistic comparison brings to light the differences and similarities between witchcraft and mediumship. The *mayabu* patient and the possessed differ not in their practice – both scream, go into trance, lose control and speak like prophets. Some patients diagnosed as having *mayabu* can later turn out to be actually suffering from a *Chwezi* affliction. Their frame of experience, though, fundamentally differs in that the healer expels the intrusion; the *Chwezi* cult embraces it. As we discover next, among Sukuma who do not belong to the cult this has led to misunderstanding.

# The Cult of Ryangombe

The history of the Chwezi dynasty has been the object of extensive research and some debate (cf. Doyle 2007; Farelius 2008). However, neither the head of the cult nor his male or female dignitaries were of any help regarding, or even seemed remotely interested in, my questions about the cult's past. Whereas members of royal dynasties usually loved to recount their history and show me lists of their ascendants, going back several centuries, none of the cult's leaders had anything written down. The songs, some containing explicit references to the mythical founder Ryangombe, simply had to speak for themselves. After all my talk about experiential structures it should not astonish the reader that what mattered to the cult leaders foremost was what the magic and the rituals could do; their experiential rather than historical significance. What counted was the place the cult and its spirits could bring participants to in the here and now. This should not, however, prevent me from indulging the reader, bracketing the *Chwezi* spirit for a while to sketch some historical contours.

Comparing myths, initiation rites, and historical records of migration and chieftaincy in the interlacustrine region of Central Africa, Luc de Heusch (1966: 249, 298, 362) concluded that the Rwandese, Ha and Ankole *Imandwa*, the Nyoro *Musegu*, the Rundi *Ikishegu*, the Luba *Mbudye*, as well as the Nyamwezi and Sumbwa *Swezi*, are cult spirits that have their common root in the legendary Kitara empire of the fifteenth century. Stretching from western Uganda to north-west Tanzania, this Bantu-speaking empire was governed by a people since relegated to mythic memory – the Chwezi, famed in the area as the founders of sacred kingship. The dynasty no longer exists. Archaeological evidence from the sites of Bigo and Ntusi in Uganda suggests the existence of fortresses (ibid.: 19). According to one hypothesis, the golden era of the Chwezi dynasty was abruptly brought to an end when Hinda (a subgroup of Luo), Nilotic invaders from the north, took advantage of internal conflicts over royal succession and invaded Kitara to chase out King Wamara. The Hinda are said to have massacred the Chwezi people, who fled with their king to the south. Mythical lore in the interlacustrine region, addressing the trauma of defeat and genocide, recounts how the survivors threw themselves in the lakes and

217

volcanoes, and since that day visit the initiated as spirits (ibid.: 37). In one version of the myth, the last Chwezi king transferred his cattle to his brother Ryangombe, who, after the invasion, founded a spirit cult within which rebels would regularly gather around the erythrine tree, symbolizing both royalty and immortality (Bösch 1930: 202). Still today, Ryangombe is acknowledged by the cult as the founder.

The antagonism between Hinda and Chwezi, respectively rulers and future cult members, prefigured a tension within the Sukuma medico-political network that would later surface, and which I heard about through my interviews with members of the royal clan of Bulima chiefdom: before Independence in the 1960s chiefs were ambivalent about the numerous medicinal associations in the villages where commoners could climb the ladder through gifts to eventually become called 'chiefs' (*batemi*) or 'kings' (*bakingi*) themselves. This ambivalence may be mutual, since Sukuma healers, on one of the rare occasions when their speech becomes historical (albeit in the form of an incantation), refer to King Luhinda both as the classificatory founder of chieftaincy and as the origin of evil to whom the healer's rites of expulsion return the curse (see also Chapter 9).

To learn about the *imandwa* spirits in Rwanda, de Heusch relied on Cory's (1955) account of *Chwezi* initiation in north Tanzania (pronounced and written *Swezi* in the south). In 1997, 2000 and 2003 I found a still vibrant *Chwezi* group close to the village in which I lived.

# The Experiential Shift

Before anyone becomes a medium they have been a patient, mostly struggling with their personal guiding ancestor. The spirit's desire for acknowledgment is manifested in a cluster of symptoms including infertility, inexplicable tiredness, chronic pains, lack of zest for living, frightening dreams, hearing voices, insomnia, autistic or uncontrolled behaviour. The news of a mediumistic vocation rarely comes as a surprise as it terminates a long therapeutic journey. The ancestor's wish, or the diviner's interpretation, may in the end be the patient's wish too, but the family will not always welcome the initiation. There are costs, such as the gift of a cow to the initiatory teacher and the transfer of three goats and the equivalent of a fourth in money to the cult's regional leaders (*bakingi*) and lower-ranked district chiefs (*batemi*), who divide the proceeds among the membership. Like all Sukuma cults, *Chwezi* members nourish solidarity and will help the initiated to gain back some of the investment later. But the cult also has to cope with negative stereotypes among the larger population.

In town I heard Sukuma speak of *Chwezi* cult members as 'witches' (*balogi*). There were rumours of public coitus during initiation, a large dose of secrecy, obscene language, strong black magic, and stories of robbers who succumbed after finding the *shishingo* diadem, a sign of *Chwezi* membership, in their loot. In the village these traits evoke the figure of the dancer rather than the witch. However, despite respect for the *Chwezi* healing tradition, there too I came across reservations. Much of the *Chwezi* initiation takes place at night. This is like an invitation to witches. What probably bothers outsiders most is that the *Chwezi* cult does not domesticate the dead, something healers normally attempt to do through sacrifice and the construction of ancestral altars.

What are *Chwezi* mediums up to with those intrusive forces? The cult answers in travel songs echoing across the valley at dusk when members walk to an event. The lyrics reassure the public that the cult of Ryangombe aims to heal, like *Lungu* and *Cheyeki* groups do, and thus actually outclasses other widely accepted groups such as *Goyangi* (snake charmers) and *Nunguli* (porcupine hunters) specializing in dance and magical combat: 'Let me subsume those two cults of pacification, *Lungu* and *Cheyeki*, under my cool ones. Ryangombe! Ryangombe! The *Goyangi* and the *Nunguli*, and the *Beeni*? Not those, they only perform dances. They do not heal people.' The song refers to the longstanding tradition of appeasement (*maholelo*). Comparing a wide range of precolonial rituals, Tcherkézoff (1985) has demonstrated that the Sukuma and their southern neighbours, the Nyamwezi, share a tradition of symbolic expulsion of the dead.[2] The song's reference to appeasement conceals from the public that the *Chwezi* differ from this tradition in not expelling the dead but 'taking care of' (*ku-langhana*) them. The cult's anthem makes no secret about it: 'Mediumship never dies. If it did, it would be like the ancestor dying today' (*Bumanga butashilaga. Bushila, ilelo isamva lyushila*).[3] Nobody can be cured of spirit mediumship (*bumanga*). The medium's special connection with the dead is for life. The *Chwezi* cult offers an alternative to cure through a cosmology and philosophy of life quite of its own.

219

Repeated in an entrancing tone, these words establish a distinction between the experience of therapy – the patient's symptoms equal the spirit's anger, which will disappear after the descendant recognizes them (cf. Chapter 2) – and the experience of possession, which refers to a life-long, mediumistic disposition. Initiation does more than expel, but is not yet the alternative to therapy envisaged by the anthem. As we will see presently, the 'reached' novice is handed over to a complex agency no ritual can command. *Chwezi* candidates therefore wear a bracelet called 'mind-broadener', *ngalike*, from the verb *kugalika*, 'to broaden (or change) one's mind'. It is one of the more direct local references to the broadening out from one experiential structure to several between which the initiate can be shifting.

## 'Dropping the Reached One'

The head of the *Chwezi* society, Ng'wana Kapini, was a difficult person to approach. But he lived in a village nearby and knew about me and Paulo from the *ihane* meetings we had attended in the area. In an interview I recorded he discussed the different stages of the *Chwezi* ritual, holding back what the cult considers secret. He knew my intentions were to publish. Our interview dictates the data I present here. When he told us that some people enter the cult for the strong protective medicine called *lushilo*, 'the end', because of its capacity to end all witchcraft, Paulo assured him that we were of that kind. During the year we had worked together there had been a number of incidences, such as illness in Paulo's family, which had been attributed to witchcraft, so our eagerness to join the cult did not surprise anyone. An initiation ceremony had already been planned for the next month. Ng'wana Kapini would notify us of the council's decision. A few weeks later we received the good news.

One evening after the harvest in 1997, the *Chwezi* party arrived on foot at our home, singing and drumming. Their number and conduct were impressive. They simply took over our compound and intervened in the ongoing household activities. There were neither greetings nor rules of reserve. Gone was the reciprocity involved in hospitality that I had been used to with guests. Those who did greet me called me 'of the big vagina' (*ng'wa ninyo*) and used *ntombo* (coitus) to mean *ntondo* (tomorrow). Paulo and I were made fools of, not taken seriously in our own home. We had become novices, denuded of accountability. The young guards (*bashilikale*), especially, were adept at keeping up the unique ambience of what to us seemed transgressive. They also kept the group in tune by playing the drums, to which dancing elders joined in at will. The guards are men and women elected for the occasion to carry spears and to wear the cult's characteristic *shishingo* diadem all through the ceremonial period while respecting the food taboos of fish, beans and sweet potatoes.

On the first day the novices are abducted and brought to the hamlet of the leading cult elder, addressed as Malamala, 'the completing one'. Just after sunset the guards circumscribe and protect the initiatory grounds against sorcery, without which, it is said, witches would take advantage of the vulnerability of the ritual's participants. The protective medicine named 'the end' is inserted inside and around the homestead. 'The end' keeps at bay everyday magical attacks. Undressed and blindfolded with a leopard skin, the leader of the guards kneels on the ground, digs a hole with his spear at the *shigiti*, a small tree-shaped constellation of medicinal vessels, and burns 'the end' with a bundle of dried long grass. About every thirty feet, the guard inserts the black concoction in the ground outside the fence. A magically circumscribed space is created within which all is safe.

From the first night the most talented mediums engage in a mastered form of trance in the public space of the cult's compound, accompanied by singing or drumming. Meanwhile, novices move inside the house. During possession the *Chwezi* spirits are asked to announce their name and, if possible, to express their demands. The 'meaningless growling' (*ku-lunduma*) of the novice has to mature into words. In an analogy with learning drum and dance patterns, the newcomers start by mimicking what they perceive, eventually entering into synchrony with the rest. Until sunrise, for five days in a row, the sultry air of the hut is filled with singing interrupted by spontaneous possessions. Bodies jam-packed together, the novices are 'reached by the ancestor' (*wa-shikilwa n'isamva*). The following song significantly depicts possession as a reciprocal process of spying on the spirits, who themselves are busy stalking the novices. 'Stalking the stalker' (*ukusuutila lusuutila*) is feeling in synchrony with what intrudes. How else could a spirit arrive, something that cannot be commanded?

| | |
|---|---|
| *Nguno ya mahugi?* | The reason for the call? |
| *Nene ili isamva nalibinishiwa lya shibyalile shane.* | I have been played upon by an ancestral spirit of my lineage. |
| *Hangi, wigele ungi, nani wa kulunduma sagala, wa ku ngw' igunga, kilinda buhile.* | If another appears, one of meaningless growling, then you should wait until it is ripe. |
| *Tugemage, mulanoga ukusuutila Lusuutila. Nene natonga.* | Let's try, before you all become tired of stalking the stalker. I go first. |

Shaking shoulders and low-pitched cries (*ku-huma*) signal the commencement of spirit possession. The spirit announces itself as a 'great snake' (*liyoka*). Sukuma understand by 'the snake' the spine, which harbours the 'life principle' and will lodge the medium's incoming spirit. Convulsions start in the spine. The spine urges the novice to dance, which can spill over into possession.

| | |
|---|---|
| *Liyoka lya maholelo likwisengaga ulu gwabala ung'weeji.* | The great cooling snake emerges when the moon appears. |
| *Likunenhelaga amang'weeshi ng'weeshi uku ngongo.* | It instils pains in my back. |
| *Mumho lyazunyaga.* | Maybe it has accepted. |

The medium depends on the snake's goodwill and on the lunar cycle. Soon the novices learn that something more than the expulsion of evil is going on. They are told to 'take care of' (*ku-langhana*) their spirit, to give it attention and cultivate a sense of timing. The medium's coinciding with an intruder left untamed is an alternative to remedies seeking to pacify. The travel song's emphasis on pacification makes it clear that the cult does not expect the uninitiated public to grasp the quaternary structure behind *Chwezi* experience. The risk in singing about the alternative to cure is, given the popular opposition of social order and witchcraft, that one becomes categorized by outsiders as a witch.

To understand, we first needed to be 'reached' and 'dropped' into a seance to assess the extent of our *Chwezi* vocation. During the interview the Malamala had surprised Paulo and me by placing all his emphasis on this opening ceremony the day after arrival. *Kugwisha mshishi* means 'causing the reached to fall'. We were told that the condition for healing is fulfilled once the initiand has lost consciousness, which Sukuma describe as 'the heart falling'. The spirits feel recognized and thus their anger recedes, and with it the descendant's symptoms. (Only after involuntary possession does the possibility of controlled mediumship arise.) As in the contingent 'yes' or 'no' of an oracle, it suffices that an extra-human presence is experienced. Then, as the Malamala told us: 'The reached ones smile. They are healed because we got hold of them'. Once the spirit has been let in, the four to seven days of rites that follow are 'just rounding off'. In other words, the frame of mediumship, experiencing synchrony with intrusion, is more important than the rites and expulsions following.

Both in divination and in *ihane* ceremonies, the checking of ancestral presence on a chicken's spleen had been a solemn occasion. But now, in dropping the reached one, our own body was going to be the oracle, deciding on the value of the ritual. Many *Chwezi* songs warn about faking possession: 'If you are pretending, oh, it will destroy you. People will say it is plain madness' (*Ulu wita makaala, yi, lyukupilingitya. Buyuhaya lilusalo*). Before the event, the fairly young master of ceremonies (*kanumba*) had a word with Paulo and me. He ordered us to take the first two turns. When the time was ripe, he said, we had to fall down on the ground, even if there was no actual possession taking place. He gave the same advice to another novice, whose turn would come after us. Apparently the most pronounced cases of mediumship were kept for the end of the ceremony. Thinking back to the song's warning, the three of us seemed rather destined for 'plain madness'. But perhaps he had underestimated how much the general ambience had affected all of us, thanks to the supportive attitude of our teachers and fellow novices, the sparkles of ecstasy that had filled the air since the previous night, and the reassuring observation that, irrespective of seniority or rank, some Chwezi members are more adept at spirit possession than others.

After the rank holders had divided the meat and beer offered by the novices, it was time for each of us to take our turn and step out of the circle where we had been waiting in the hot afternoon sun. All attention was on the novice led into the darkness of the house and placed on the traditional round stool to become *mshishi*, a 'reached one', derived from the verb *ku-shisha*, 'to make arrive'. I cannot help pointing to the similarity with the etymology of 'contingency', the arrival of the real in divination.

223

The stool, low and encompassing the buttocks, refers to the ancestor, both as a source of authority (the word 'stool', *isumbi*, is used for 'rank') and as a transitional space between life and the grave (remember the stool is split during burial). To protect the possessed in their vulnerable state of receptivity, a black concoction is smeared on top of the head, the inside of the forearms, the chest, armpits and under the feet. Closely encircled by teacher and disciples, the candidate clenches a tiny bundle of dried long grass in both hands at chest height. A wooden stick supports the feet. In this way the body remains in suspension, separated from the ground and demarcated by the two main constituents of the bush in their sapless state: a log of wood and a bundle of cut grass, two natural materials which, besides recalling death and regeneration, represent the two main ranks of power in Sukuma societies (*ngogo* and *sanzu*, respectively). The intention of the rite – attraction of the spirit – is expressed in a string of small branches of the plant called *luduta*, 'the pulling' (from *ku-duta*, to pull), and tied around the novice's stool. To further attract the spirit, a *shishingo* diadem, containing the secret root of mediumship, is held above the fontanelle. The 'climbing' (*kubuula*) of the ancestral spirit commences as the teacher sounds a small portable drum twice at the forehead, fontanelle and back. The small space of the hut is packed with singing, drumming and rattling disciples calling up the ancestor, enclosing more and more upon the novice. The incantations, rattle shakes and drumming intensify once the novice gives the impression of losing control, the shoulders shaking to rhythmic, ever-louder, higher-pitched growls. 'Nyabalenge, you become like a bow straightening' (*Nyabalenge, ubangile buta ukangoola*), the song summons over and over again. The 'reached one' gradually leans backwards until falling to the ground. The drumming stops and the novice screams or speaks. Assistants then carry this person to a room next door, where his or her name is repeated until consciousness is regained.

Just like the others, I found myself in that room, repeating my name to the teacher's question 'Who are you? Did we do you wrong?' I was confused and could not stand up immediately. My legs and arms felt numb and I had to hit them to get the blood circulating again and raise myself. Paulo asked me what had happened. When I staggered out of the house, I became aware of a sharp pain in the left temple. There was a marked swelling. I could not remember whether my head had actually touched the ground while leaning backwards.

In the central courtyard sounded a song to welcome 'the reached ones' that we had learned the previous night.

| | |
|---|---|
| *Baba, unene nilabilaga, ng'wana Bugeke, nabahila.* | Father, look at me, child of Bugeke, I have spoken in voices. |
| *Banhu bakasalaga. Watushiga, umani wa mazwanoge, watuleka.* | People are going mad. He has left us, the expert of medicine, he left us to ourselves. |
| *Bukuyombaga uboongo. Untwe gwasebile. Lwabi lwane.* | The mind goes on speaking. The head has been mingled with. It has become mine. |
| *Waibuta inghingi iyo yanijamyaga.* | You have cut the king post that supported me. |
| *Waibuta imbeho iyo nikingijaga.* | You have cut the shade that protected me. |
| *Iki naluha. Bupina buluhi.* | Therefore I am suffering. Tormenting sorrow. |

Once 'dropped', we were barely given time to recover. As mere vehicles of the deceased, the novices are at this stage treated like animals. Crawling over the ground and chased by the guards, we were ordered to repeat our morning routine of licentious verses: 'The thing got stuck going into the anus', 'The clitoris drops by lack of lovers', and 'The sun is burning. Let's plant lentils in the vagina'. An ambience of threat and uncertainty ruled. We were prohibited to stand up or wash our hands before eating the few unpeeled sweet potatoes that the cooks had reserved for us. Lying on the ground, hungry and deprived of shade, we stared at the *Chwezi* cult members enjoying their meals and once in a while throwing picked bones at our feet. Nothing more was needed for us to long for the next phase of the ritual which would enable us to end the condition in which we found ourselves, and regain the consciousness lost.

# Regaining the Senses

The morning after the rite of *kugwisha*, which had confirmed everyone's possession by *Chwezi* spirits, we burned the bundle of grass that our fists had clenched during the séance and ran in circles spreading the smoke in the central courtyard. This smoke was our spirit, we were told. Then we spoke and sang in the obscene metaphors that had been taught to us the previous days.

Unaccomplished mediums are dangerously 'hot' (*basebu*). On bare feet and with head bent, each of us approached the centre of the compound, where the master of ceremonies sat on the traditional stool covered with a leopard skin and tied with the 'pulling' plant. He weaved the plant into *lubuha* bracelets and smeared them with the blood of a sacrificed goat and three types of protective medicine. Then he tied one around each novice's neck as well as on the left or right wrist and ankle, depending on whether the spirit imposing its call belonged to the paternal or maternal clan. In the coming days the bracelet would itch, smell of blood, and attract swarms of flies. The bracelet binds the carriers to a *Chwezi* ancestor, but also protects them against the sorcery to which they are vulnerable when leaving the space circumscribed by 'the end'. Together with a hundred or so initiated *Chwezi* and *Chwengele* (a sub-group),[4] the thirty-two of us lined up to cross 'the outside' (*ibaala*) and meander through the fields to reach the forest.

In half a day, until sunset, we covered all the stages of 'the big forest' (*bu ng'hale*) where 'secrets' (*mabanga*) were taught. The teachers completed the training sessions by anointing our bodies with the black residues of burnt groundnuts, as dry and earthly as death. Before that, we had come to appropriate the chief plant of the cult ritually. It suffices to say that its outlook and name refer to immortality and to the correct term for greeting a king. A month earlier, King Kaphipa of Bukumbi chiefdom had recounted to me how he had been installed as king fifty years ago. His father's dignitaries had abducted him at night to bury him alive. They were, in his words, acting like sorcerers. A commoner could become king through a subversion of social order, whereby death, evil and sorcery were incorporated rather than expelled. The *Chwezi* novices are also abducted to perform a subversion of the social order. Could the enthronement ceremony of the old *Chwezi* dynasty have been an inspiration? In any case, transformation was the grand notion with which we left the forest feeling uplifted and we sang the medium's anthem about ancestors lifting their curse while our newly found state of mediumship would never die.

The ritual stage of the 'big forest' helps the novices to overcome their inhibition over embracing the announcing spirit, an inhibition understandable from the Sukuma aversion to loss of self-control (for which I have seen Pentecostalists ridiculed on market days). As the next song reveals, once the gaze of the other no longer inhibits, nothing can stand in the way between the medium and their fate.

| | |
|---|---|
| *Baana baneye, nalekelwa izumo.* | My children, I have left the curse behind. |
| *Nyanjige, nabi liiso lukuni.* | Nyanjige [a name], I have become clairvoyant. |
| *Uku nzila nduhu ihamo, uku Welelo.* | On the road lies nothing, but fate. |
| *Ukubyala, namala. Ninga.* | To give birth, I finished. I have come out. |
| *Ukusekwa na banhu. Nabi liiso lukuni.* | To be laughed at by people. I have become clairvoyant. |

The next day teacher and novice spend together in making the *shishingo* diadem from the root of the cult's chief plant. On the root the teacher sows several rows of cowries, their base opening vertically, like female genitals, and towards the sky. The black tail of a bushbuck antelope (*mbushi*) is connected to the back. Thus the pupil obtains an oblong diadem extending from the middle of the forehead to the fontanelle (*manda*), where the spirit enters before descending to the spine.

During the fourth night, the ritual procedures followed on from each other closely. First the teachers made an end to our unaccomplished ritual condition (*kumelamela*). In the pitch dark we were brought to an intersection, where each novice sat on the ancestral seat and received medicinal incisions on the chest and on top of the head. The teacher then turned his back on the pupil. His two little fingers reaching for the pupil's, the latter was lifted up while his or her right foot toppled a cooking pot covered with a jackal hide. In *ihane*, too, this movement signified the accomplishment of initiation.

The teacher addressed the novice with the words *walijiwa badugu*. The probable translation is: 'you have been fed the ancestors'. To eat is an ominous expression, referring to occult appropriation, but not within the *Chwezi* frame. Healing becomes a life-long journey, one that even the Malamala, the 'completing one', admits never having finished:

| | |
|---|---|
| *Bebe, Lyang'ombe. Twakufuha ubebe iki welaga.* | You, Ryangombe. We aspersed you, for you shine brightly. |
| *Tulekelage amabaala gose tugidinge.* | Let's desert all places to roam freely. |
| *Tutumame unimo ugo walutumamaga.* | Let us do the work as you did before us. |
| *Tuhoje banhu pye. N'unene ukanihoje.* | Let us heal all people. And may you heal me. |

With their former selves dead, the newly initiated are ready to regain their senses. This must be taken literally. They move into the forest (*ku mabuga*), this time at night, to consecutively taste the spirit, smell medicinal vapours, and feel on their skin the soil of the ancestors. At a termite mound, which represents the ancestral realm, they first make a vow on the tomb of their cult parents and grandparents. Then, lying down at a tunnel dug at the base of the termite-mound, they wait for Ng'wana Kapini to take a mouthful of flour mixture and asperse them. Still lying down, the newly initiated drink from the water at the base of the termite mound, thus ingesting the ancestor. They perform the opposite of aspersions placating the ancestors. Each of the *Chwezi* seniors chooses a novice as their child. Parents and children then make gestures as if copulating, which, in 'the spirit' of the cult, is not a transgression of the incest prohibition but a negation of the existence of that prohibition. They act as spirits do when possessing. Then the tunnel is destroyed and the group returns to the compound in a euphoric state. They have performed 'convulsions in the forest' (*kugalagala mu bu*). Preparations are underway for the two final stages of the therapy: fumigation (*luhiga*) and mud massage (*lutaka*).

Small groups of patients take turns around a pot of medicinal water dug into the ground. Boiling-hot hearthstones are dropped in the pot and a large cloth is placed over groups of patients inhaling the steam released. Soon after, the heat is alternated with the utter coldness of a mud massage. For the rest of the night the patients dance topless in a circle while being covered all over with fresh mud, made of cow dung, wet soil and herbs. The other members help them through this ordeal with moral support, songs and drumming. *Chwezi* initiands compare the mud to the flour mixture with which healers asperse their ancestral altars. (Moreover, some clans are known to smear mud on their ancestral altars.) On top of the bodily sensation of contrast, the mud massage thus has the effect of transforming the medium into an altar for the ancestor.

By sunrise the initiands, shivering with cold, line up to leave the ritual space of the compound. At the exit each of them jumps over a black cloth covering the master of ceremonies who had tied their *luduta* bracelets. From there the whole group continues down to a pond to bathe (*ha lyoga*) and collect their diadem from the *shigiti* tree, which stood in the central courtyard. The Malamala pronounces the final formula:

| | |
|---|---|
| *Abakoyiwagwa Buchwezi, twabumalaga.* | Those who had Chwezi trouble, we ended that. |
| *Bahole, babyale, bitombe, bapone, basabe, balagule.* | Let them heal, give birth, have sex, harvest, get rich, cure [others]. |

Guards accompany the novice home, where millet stalks (*ibelele*) inserted in the roof and an altar of 'remainders' (*misagati*) will remind them of a small follow-up ceremony to be held at a later date. The little round construction of wooden sticks diverging towards the sky perfectly inverts the domesticating inclination of the clan's own ancestral altar, which closes on top.

## Therapy and Subversive Structure

Though stretching over five days, the initiation followed the chronology of a day-long cycle: at sunset the blindfolded magician demarcates the ritual space; at noon the initiands are dropped into a symbolic void to reach the spirit; in the afternoon and at night they regain their senses; at sunrise their new life commences. This (classic) dialectic of rebirth unfolds in tension with possession proper: the unpredictable moments when the spirit overtakes one, mostly at night. Equally indicative is the contrast with *ihane* village initiation into the society of elders. There the young men become accredited as 'feathers of the Sukuma wing', to obey the laws of clan and community so that ancestral spirits inhabit the domestic altars and do not roam freely. In contrast, *Chwezi* initiation does not stimulate the slightest interest in reintegrating spirits, let alone the novices, into village life. The cult typically negates gender division and village rules, desiring that the mediums do 'roam freely' as in the last song. The *Chwezi* altar opens up towards the sky, whereas the domestic altars of the ancestors converge. While the *ihane* novices leave the village and enter the forest to return empowered at the house's threshold, the spirit mediums progressively spiral outwards to the pond at the periphery of the village. No better example of opposite structures of experience within one and the same culture.

Bugeke's child, in the song, had her protective shade 'cut'. Her support, the house's king post (associated with the father), had fallen apart. She suffered and sang that 'the mind goes on speaking'. But 'it has become mine', she added, opting for the shock of possession as a way of life. She discovered a logic that, unlike the protective *lushilo* medicine Paulo and I went for, really sets an 'end' to the dialectic of social redress sustained by ritual healing. *Chwezi* initiates learn that people normally enjoy social order, that bewitchment may breach it, that the order can be restored through remedy, but that possession is neither of these three.

She would live on with her *shishingo* diadem, as it opens up to the spirit and connects her to a world without prohibitions or selves to feel guilty or envious about. Could this position 'beyond therapy' (hence beyond social redress) explain the sense of superiority I know many mediums to combine with their tragic state of affliction? The moment of possession, of the spirit entering, is all sacrifice and no gift. Our table of cultural comparison (Figure 4.1) had a place for sacrifice without gift, namely the fourth column, the one experiential frame we have not discussed so far. Spirit possession has no place with magic (second column: reciprocity) nor with ritual sacrifice (third column: expulsion). It concerns intrusion but deals with it in a manner opposite to the first column, which 'totalizes', in the sense of submits, the total system to one calculus, that of transaction. Spirit possession is unpredictable, pure sacrifice.

Yet, initiation into the spirit can be therapeutic. Entering the spirit world is to stimulate the participant's capacity of alternating experiential frames and having these structures coexist. On the last day of initiation I casually conversed with a fellow participant who had been unable to utter a word the week before. I speculate that even severe psychical disorders can benefit from the subversion of *Chwezi* initiation. Chapter 2 touched on Bateson's (1990: 190) definition of schizophrenia as the inability to set meta-communicative frames and to take metaphors other than literally. Teasing such multiple structures back into the novice's picture, do the *Chwezi* rites not replicate, in a more refined way, the psychotic's survival reflex of hallucinatory perception?

Spirits exhibit, for all to see, the discontinuity between experience and culture. If their hint at individual freedom is 'subversive' and seems to contradict local conceptions of sociality, it is precisely because possession is exceptional, rather than representative of society, and because it concerns the very crisis of that sociality. A study in terms of experiential frames allows for a dynamic understanding of culture that can account for an individual's shift of experience without having to surmise cultural contradiction.

The subversive nature of the experiential shift shows in the cult's breach of Sukuma conventions. Sexual segregation is suspended. Men and women wash together, sit and eat together. Conversations freely explore otherwise restricted themes such as comparisons of male and female sexuality. The cult's activities disregard clan and village life where public release of emotion is unacceptable. The pinnacle of this is perhaps the symbolic denial of the incest taboo. The subversion of social distinctions is a permanent feature of the *Chwezi* cult rather than the pivot in a ritual dialectic. Whereas the dancer's violation of social order takes place between the brackets of an appropriate space-time (every Sukuma is a dancer at some point in their life), the possessed lives out crisis, involving a loss of self, which they embrace just as society would be screaming for redress. The pure sacrifice to the spirit decentres both self and society. What can easily be downplayed as inversion by a binary code (social order versus disorder, or reason versus emotion) can appear, thanks to our quaternary table, to be subversion.

It should be clear that by subversion I mean a type of experiential structure rather than a particular belief or line of thought. The latter would make me vulnerable to Janet McIntosh's recent 'counterpoint to those studies that celebrate possession's subversive overtones' (McIntosh 2004: 92). She challenges Boddy's (1989) thesis on embodied counter-hegemony with the fact that Giriama spirits in Kenya embody Muslim hegemony, whose oppression of local beliefs is lamented in interviews only after the seance. Still, McIntosh's observation of (involuntary) possessions by a reprimanding Muslim spirit confirms that the message staged is an experience of crisis, otherwise left inarticulate. Her counter-example displays the structure of subversion. We are still in the situation of a person giving voice to an intrusive, moral power that one prefers not to talk about in public.

The night before *kugwisha* (the spirit's arrival) saw much emotional release. A *Chwengele* song about women's fate spilled over in spirit-led convulsions from the spine among several experienced mediums. The song relates the life of the bride, her suffering in the service of her household, and the bit of comfort she gets from her sisters-in-law.

| | |
|---|---|
| *Makaya malambu, baniki.* | Difficult homes, girls. |
| *Ukumona ng'wiyo, waliitenganije mpaga lyugwilwa milage, wakoyagakoyaga yii.* | To see your friend, how she empowered [the home] to the point of succumbing with the soot [of the pot], so much she suffered. |
| *Ng'wana wa bukwingwa, kanituulile wanzuki mpaga niisikie.* | Child of the wife-givers [sister-in-law], bring me honey-beer until I feel it. |

The wedding song 'Liars!' (see Chapter 3) receives its sequel here in the *Chwezi* cult. Spirit possession seems a culturally specific way of doing something universal: resisting a social condition that becomes too weighty. The same moral power that is feared by the one as a cause of death (*sengi*'s cattle of the lap) can for the other be a reality in need of articulation (the bride's chores). Sustaining personal crisis is useful here in exposing a social condition, a state of the system otherwise hidden.

At this point my analysis converges with some of the literature. Anthropology rediscovered spirit possession at a time when essentializing cultures became a thing of the past and a more globalized perspective was sought. Following the appeal of Bourdieu's (1980: 51–87) concept of practice combining socio-political conditions and culture-specific dispositions, the literature on spirit cults boomed. It introduced two paradigms that dominated the study of practices in general throughout the 1990s: power/resistance, and (therapeutic) embodiment in culture (see, e.g., Comaroff 1985; Boddy 1989; Devisch 1993). The two paradigms make sense. First, initiation into the *Chwezi* cult yields a supportive network, which raises a member's power as well as the group's influence on society. Secondly, initiation means therapy by playing on the cultural in the body and the bodily in culture.

However, heeding van Binsbergen's (2003) reflections on his *Sangoma* initiation, one may ask: what would my *Chwezi* friends think of the above analysis? In explaining spirit possession in terms of power and healing, we attribute to it the purposive action that, as

Crapanzano (1977: 29) warned, 'may very well be precluded by the spirit idiom itself '. Do such instrumentalist explanations not mean rejection of the possessed's belief in an agency of its own called spirit? The dilemma is that, if we proceed from the so-called 'fact' of spirit agency (see Willis 1999: 116; E. Turner 2004: 55), we are again in danger of objectifying the local view in the positivist terms of a truth claim. We would be placing beliefs in spirits on a par with empirical knowledge of, say, neurons. We would be misframing spirits for the reader. Considering the difference between a mediumistic and a scientific epistemology, a fairer translation of the medium's spirit in our (scientific) terms might be 'desire', as in Lienhardt's (1970) notion of spirits as *passiones*.[5] Janice Boddy's (1994) seminal review paved the way for a performative model of spirit possession, which avoids both instrumentalism and positivism. The cult, a social rather than individual body, performs the spirit for its own sake, as in art for art's sake. The ethnographer leaves open the question of subjective intentions, social consequences or the meaning of spirits.

During a meeting halfway through our initiation I witnessed a sharp discussion when someone proposed not initiating novices unable to pay the necessary fees (an anecdote mentioned in Chapter 1). A tall elder with a red shirt and a cowboy hat stood up and gained approval when he protested in a low carrying voice: 'This is not business but your ancestral spirit. There is no leader in spirit matters' (*Iti biashara, isamva lyako duhu. Ati ntale mu isamva*). He thus conveyed his awareness of logics conflicting. Had the novices come to heal, or to attain *Chwezi* status by paying a fee (hence 'business'), or because their spirit wanted it?

My answer has been: all of these. The cult occasions moments of power, intrusion, therapy and performance (synchrony with the spirit). Inspired by Jackson and Karp's (1990: 17) reference to William James's pragmatic definition of truth, I have approached the literature's paradigms not as conflicting claims of truth but as distinct frames of experience. The frames are each relevant for practices of possession, albeit at different moments. Michael Lambek (1993) has demonstrated how sorcery, Islamic religion and spirit possession coexist as three alternative forms of politico-religious knowledge and practice on the island of Mayotte. If we treat those religious forms as experiential frames, it not only appears that the distinct frames can be encountered within the spirit cult, sometimes colliding (as can be

233

gathered from the tall elder's concern), and that these frames to some extent invoke each of the alternative practices. The distinct frames can also be related within a holistic structure. This holism explains why *Chwezi* concerns are recognizable across cultures. It clarifies the distinctions made by the anthropologist. What holism loses in ethnographic specificity it gains in reflexivity.

## Notes

1.  See Stroeken (2006) for a concise literature overview.
2.  This is another good reason for calling the third frame of experience relating to divination and healing ritual 'expulsive'.
3.  I thank Pelle Brandström for taking up with me the poor translation I offered for this quote in Stroeken (2006).
4.  The *Chwengele* sub-group differs from *Chwezi* in having a smaller joining fee and fewer ceremonies, though it does have more, mostly collective, mediumistic seances.
5.  Just as spirits retain some opacity for the possessed themselves, passions and conscious experience in general remain something of a mystery to biologists. Science cannot tell us where a person's desire should ultimately be located: in neurons or in thoughts/emotions.

# Chapter 9
# Magic, Ritual and the Senses

Mashala was not a spirit medium. He was thought to suffer from a *ndagu* curse, of the *ibona* type. The problem started after he chased away his maternal aunt. She had come to stay in his compound, suffering from a reputation that, according to Mashala's mother, she did not deserve. Mashala fell ill some time after she left. He went to the district hospital in Bukumbi. He had used the best protective magic. But all of this was to no avail. The question became how to make sure that the witch's attacks stopped. How to bring to an end the grudge that she bore, now shared with her accomplices, and knowing that the reason of the witch is harsh, not that of a person listening to reason or interested in social exchange? How to end the grudge of somebody who remains secretive about it, whose identity and motives remain unfathomable to non-witches? The lethal witchcraft in magic refers to her moral power and her expertise in winning over the victim's ancestral guide. The victim got *ndagu*, literally 'the treatment'.

Diviners, whether or not trained as *Chwezi* mediums, embrace the moral power emanating from crisis in the form of a spirit, a dream or a ripened ulcer. For themselves the sense of intrusion may even be a source of pleasure and pride. But for the patient such experience is to be domesticated, its source exorcized. Rituals are occasions within the public setting of the healer's compound or the village which signal on whose side the sources of authority and power stand. The lingering conflation we called 'moral power' is drummed out in healing rites. In therapy the comforting frame that has been instigated in divination is more durably instantiated. Most divinations propose a three-fold therapy. Sacrifice (*shitambo*) of beer or goat at the altars is literally a 'hunt' for ancestral approval. Secondly, the ascendant's bracelets and amulets should reconnect the patient's body to the ancestors (a pastoralist extension, if you will). Thirdly, the body is incised, smeared or fed with herbal medicine (an agricultural intervention, if you will).

As the reader may remember from the chicken oracle discussed in Chapter 7, Mashala had improved his connection with the ancestors by wearing their bracelets. He had taken medicinal preparations enriched with ingredients dreamt up by his diviner, Seele. Her oracles had been successful in expressing the nature of his condition, which he once recounted to me as verging on *litunga*, 'tied', like his abruptly deceased and abducted sister. The metaphor of the python captures the inverted womb the abducting witch is imagined to be: not gestating but swallowing. The victim is represented in black magic by a blind puppy (*kanyanabona*). Mashala had used the counter-remedy called 'the untier', *italigula* (from *ku-taligula*, 'to untie' or 'to open'). The curative 'white' remedy is meant to untie the bad spell. The concoction is heavily rubbed all over the body with a *shilungu*, a round white shell. The red version of 'the untier' cools down the spell caused by a corrupted ancestor. The black version hides the ancestor away from the corrupting influence of the witch.

Despite the sophisticated magic, Mashala's wife lost a baby and then became sick. Something more radical was needed to treat the curse. Lukundula's son (who had in the meanwhile taken over his father's practice along with his sister Seele) saw it fit that Mashala perform a ritual of expulsion together with his two co-wives and the others of his household. The ritual would also consist of an appeasement of the ancestor at his altar. All the huts and especially the kitchen had to be ritually cleansed, since one could not exclude the possibility that a household member had conspired with the witch to corrupt the ancestor's blessing. The main issue was to denounce the witch's intervention as an evil curse and, at the same time, win over the protective ancestor of Mashala. I happened to be present as they prepared the ritual.

At dawn, a goat was chosen, the *mbuli ya ng'huba*, 'goat of lack'. The goat makes the ancestor present, just like the 'eye' on the spleen in an oracle. The goat accompanied us throughout the exorcism. Around noon, the patient and all household members gathered inside the house to be anointed with protective medicine. The medicine did not cover the whole body (as in daily medicinal massage) but targeted strategic spots, thought to be vulnerable to the witch's intrusion,

236

especially the top of the head, the centre of the chest, and the soles of the feet. (During exorcism the witch is said to easily access participants.) The household placated the ancestors by aspersing a mixture of water and flour at the base of the altars. When night fell, we went out in the pitch dark to stand at a crossroads, everyone facing west. A pit was dug between the two converging paths, into which each household member put a black concoction of counter-magic. They repeated the healer's words, verse by verse. The expulsion was visible on the facial expression and the verbal intonations of the participants. I could not help but notice the determined look on Mashala's five-year-old son's face as he confronted the illness of his mother after mourning the death of his little sister. Together, they sent the curse back to where it belongs, to the deep waters of the lake. The healer's formula ended with a standard reference to the notoriously cruel king Luhinda.

> I deploy my *ndagu* healing. Me, Ichaniki, I summon you, Ndagu, who has been convoked at my homestead and at my body. Now I expel you from my body. I leave you at this crossroads or remit you to the witch who has sent you. I expel you to the lake, so that you will be eaten by the crocodiles. Go away and die in the lake, go, grandchild of Luhinda.[1]

Then the goat's ear was cut and the blood was collected, mixed with the medicine and smeared on the spearhead held by the head of the household. Each participant had to lick the spear before the end of it was prodded into the pit. The healer made two heaps of grass and lit them while muttering words similar to the earlier incantation. The father held the goat, while the healer went around them with the burning grass. The fire was then extinguished by sticking the bundle of grass in the pit. In close formation all household members left the spot without looking back, to prevent the curse from returning. The healer stayed behind with the goat. The household members entered the hut, from whence they had started. Each was incised on head, chest and armpits, and had a protective ointment rubbed in. All thresholds and entrances were reinforced with the magic. The healer extinguished the kitchen fire by sprinkling water on it from a bundle of leaves dipped in the protective mixture. The men seized this female space, replaced the hearth stones, and rekindled both the kitchen fire and the simmering external fire (*shikome*) in the compound's central yard (*luganga*) next to the cattle pen in the traditional way rubbing sticks. Every morning, for four days, the household members smeared their entire bodies with the protective ointment. At the end of the procedure the women were visibly relieved. Mashala's son gave me a smile after I said that his mother seemed to be on the way to recovery (she was). They all, Mashala told me, left a very dark period behind them.

Ritual exorcism resembles divination in causing a shift from intrusion to expulsion. The shift applies less to diviner or healer, who may be in a state of trance, than to the other participants. The ritual actions and formulas relate to their experience. As the ancestral spirit arrives to side with the client and to help expose the witch, the cause of evil becomes an identifiable culprit, who can be beaten by stronger magic. The shift allows for concrete measures of counter-magic. What we are observing in the readiness of the patient for magical combat is not a reduction of anxiety but a radical transformation in how the body and the senses are orientated in the environment. A quick overview of the ethnography in sensorial terms should clarify this.

In the Sukuma language, possessing a thing is 'being with' it, being a companion rather than an owner (the one 'owed' to). I tried to highlight this philosophy of life that alternates gift and sacrifice. I have not shunned from calling it magical. In the village, men and women form a homestead that gains status by accumulating offspring, allies, membership in societies and medicinal knowledge, a collection that is simultaneously subject to the blessing of ancestors. The reciprocal receptivity showed in procedures of commensality and greeting, both marked by an art of stalling and patience and respect. Greetings consist of an elaborate play on sensory signals that solicit rather than command attention. Sukuma are known in the country for potions of *samba*, meant to attract from a distance. The magic is popular among a clientele as varied as dancers, prospective lovers and shopkeepers who aim to maintain a receptive attitude among clients even in the harsh domain of doing business.

*Samba* remedies are a 'red' as well as 'cool' type of medicine, situated between black (aggressive) and white (curative) magic. The term derives from *ku-samba(guka)*, 'to provoke'. The user's objective is to become popular or desired. A common kind of *samba* involves licking the red powder of the *nkulungu* tree and smearing it on one's molars. Another kind is a foamy concoction of red roots of the *nkaanya* tree, which become prickly and self-catalysing after grinding, giving a busy impression. These ground roots are mixed with millet stalks (*ibelele lya busiga*). Several other medicines are ranked within the category of *samba*. *Ihumuja* (from *ku-humula*, 'to be quiet') is a popular medicine by which all present become silent when the user speaks. *Masabiile* serves to keep opponents in a dance competition stuck to their dancing spot. *Ngweshi* (from *ku-gwesa*, 'to pull') is used to attract clients for business. A medicine bordering on the illicit is *lukomolo* (from *ku-komola*, 'to change one's mind') used to prejudice one's sexual partner. Its *shingila*, 'access', is the partner's earwax, which according to my informant establishes a double metonymic link, one to the identity of the victim and the other to the magical aim of blocking the ears. This non-lethal magic resembles *lemaga* (from *ku-lema*, 'to refuse') which makes the victim stubbornly deny all treatment. I have more than once heard reference to *lemaga* when an elder, thought to be bewitched by his wife, refused protective medicine. Enjoying bewitchment is a genuine possibility. Not only with love potions. Even with magic of aggressive intent the experiential frame of its application is reciprocal: the herbs and other ingredients establish an exchange between the home (*kaya*) and the curative forces from the forest (*bu*).

Reciprocal receptivity, or 'being with', resembles the 'dwelling' perspective that Ingold (2000) observed among Arctic hunters. He contrasted this with the 'building' perspective of analytical reason categorizing the world which Westerners specialize in. From my data on bewitchment and divination it appears that one should be careful to exclude people from this building perspective – that is, from pure reason. There may be different occasions for different perspectives on the world, and these differences in perspective within one and the same culture may even go deep, right down to the senses. Social situations alter the way of perceiving our environment. That quality of sensory perception can be understood as cross-cutting our sensory modes, such as vision, hearing, touch and so on. This book has dealt with structures of experience. The two components can be further specified. Experience comprises sensory perception. Frame or structure includes orderings and codes. In the following my analysis delves into the sensory dimension of both structure and experience. I return to the question of why and how magic works (see Chapter 2). As the interface of mind and body, the senses seem particularly liable to interconnect widely separate parts of the system and be the pivot for meaningful actions that improve an organism's homeostasis.

Sukuma practices know more sensory codes than 'being with'. Faced with affliction or misfortune, people construct witches that are no longer tricksters or dancers but envious secretive others, endowed with surprisingly moral overtones reminiscent of provoked ancestors. Shaped by the concrete, sensory experience of affliction, the construct of the witch reflects the pain and intrusion the patient physically experiences. The sensory code crosscuts several sensory modes. The sensory intrusion is cognized in suspicions about an absolute outsider within. 'You will see my revenge'. Receptive vision becomes intrusive. Nocturnal sounds become invasive. Food ingested days before acquires a poisonous aftertaste. Touch can be felt as intrusive, hiding ulterior motives. Not only the exteroceptive senses (perception external to the body) are requalified. Patients attend to the slightest interoceptive changes. The poison of bewitchment may be felt in the stomach. The bird's entrails reveal this poison. 'Being with' has perverted into a permeable body invaded by the witch.

Divination starts from this feeling. It takes a critical look at the world and thereby establishes its wretched state in terms of unreliable ancestors and envy, and the desire among kin to kill other kin. This need to identify evil is very different from the attempt to live with the uncertainties of life. Indeed, the oracular signs and categories have much in common with the representational perspective that, according to Ingold (ibid.: 168), marks the dominant Western scientific code of looking. The bewitched seems to perceive the world devoid of the ancestor's soothing influence, a world in which debts are fixed and people categorized. The intrusive code of perception, which comes close to the representational perspective Ingold attributes to modern science, is thus also found among the Sukuma, but only in times of crisis.

Diviners and healers operate a third code of vision, one that refers to the presence of the ancestral spirit in oracles. The 'eye' of ancestral presence encapsulates clients and healers in a reassuring, centripetal relationship with authority. I have suggested that this instantiation of the eye has therapeutic effects. Lévi-Strauss (1972; see Chapter 6) claimed that metaphors render pain tolerable through externalization. Most commentaries have agreed with the social and psychic effectiveness of shamanic healing, but, being wedded to a Cartesian dichotomy between meaning and matter, have rejected any physiological effects as fantasy: metaphors belong in the domain of meaning (Neu 1975: 285). In contrast, I argue that shifts between sensory codes are meaning-initiated physiological events. Paving the way for future work, this final chapter explores how sensory shifts might heal; and how healers may thus dispose of a proper knowledge, one of a transmodal kind.

The above sensory codes form a neat ternary cycle of reciprocity, breach, and redress maintaining the status quo. To break out of the cycle, spirit possession takes away the reason for feeling intruded upon. Mediums are after the spirit who is after them. Mediumship is an alternative to healing. In more than one way, also sensorily, the *Chwezi* spirit cult can be considered a terminal point, or an 'ending' (*lushilo*) as the cult's magical recipe is fittingly called. A man blindfolded with leopard skin uses *lushilo* to circumscribe the cult's ritual space. Within this circle 'ends' the power of the envious witch and the power of village norms. The cult members are blind to society's distinctions of gender, age and kinship. They no longer have reason to gain status, 'collect' and 'be with' others (the first sensory code of reciprocal receptivity), nor to fear debt, guilt, envy and witchcraft (the second sensory code of intrusion), nor to combat the witch and redress the capacity to engage in social exchange (the third sensory code of expulsion). The fourth sensory code differs from the other three codes in that the self of the possessed seeks to synchronize with the other (a spirit) rather than reciprocate or be with it, feel intruded upon by it, or do away with it. The blindfold evokes this state of utter receptivity, labelled in Figure 4.1 as 'pure sacrifice'. The blindfold does not take away vision, nor does it render categorization impossible. The senseless cries or silence of the possessed should not fool us: the *Chwezi* novices discover another way of seeing, another way of categorizing the world. Blindfold is a fourth code of vision complementary and opposite to the trio of glance, intrusive look and eye. These four complementary opposites could have headed our table of social exchange. The experiential is as much social, and vice versa. Therefore, magic works.

241

# Synaesthetics: The Art and Technology of Magic

Simply put, the principle of Sukuma magic is that meaning heals the body. This formula has to be read in a non-Cartesian way, namely without separating matter and meaning. In biomedical terms the message reads: not only matter heals. The role of non-biological factors in improving health will come hardly as a surprise. Scientists today acknowledge that meanings stimulating psychological and social harmony contribute to recovery. A more challenging cultural difference comes to light if we consider how healers conceive of these meanings. They categorize ingredients conveying a meaning as forms of 'access', *shingila*. Besides curative plants that physically affect the patient, the magical recipe also contains ingredients that physically affect by communicating meanings both to the users themselves (who have been initiated to prepare the medicine) and to the natural and social environment they work in. Those ingredients are supposed to find the gateway to the sensory shifts we discussed.

It may be astonishing that Sukuma healers found it necessary to invent such a duality of ingredients, which goes back to at least the early 1940s when Cory (1949) did his research: the medicinal plants (roots, bark, leaves) on the one hand and the 'access' on the other. It looks like an attitude more open and comprehensive than the one-sidedly materialistic paradigm of modern medicine. This comprehensive duality in fact rejects the classic idea of a non-Cartesian attitude of users of magic, for whom there would be no such separate thing as matter; for whom meaning in itself is sufficient to effect healing. So where does the well-informed addition of meaning to matter come from? Clients told me that healers make a big deal about the second category, 'access', and justify their payment by referring to it. Could that more creative part be a source of business and thus be cleverly mystified by them, especially since many of the first category, the plants, are common knowledge? There is more to it, I argue. A more detailed example will illustrate that communication with the environment is intrinsic to magical recipes. The recipes are structured linguistically, like composite words. Access is their purpose, and for healers and patients this is a veridical notion. As the reader will have noticed by now, both parties want to see results, and engage in trial and error to achieve this purpose.

Collective rituals such as fertility ceremonies at the start of cultivation involving the whole village in a transformative process are, to my knowledge, no longer practised in this part of the world. However, people engage in all sorts of rituals at home or in a cult, ranging from public rites, such as *ihane* initiation, to more discrete ones, such as expulsive rites and the application of magic. Here I illustrate the latter kind.

Before sowing his fields, Paulo decided to perform a ritual of protection, which he had learned from his brother. To protect his crops against thieves and witches, he roasted some maize seeds in a black potsherd. The black colour and the potsherd evoke lethal counter-attack. The roasted seeds were mixed with a tiny piece of elephant trunk, the latter referring to the imagined culprit such as a thief or other intruder the magic protects against (in the old days elephants plundered people's maize fields). After grinding the seeds Paulo poured water that had been standing in his house for a few days. With the concoction he drew a cross at the threshold of his house. He anointed the maize seeds and poured the pile in a bowl placed on a *lugobi* ring meant for carrying loads on the head and made of weeds that grow at intersections. He undressed, put on his ancestral amulet and carried the bowl on his head and sneaked out to his fields.

Step by step he adopted the same procedure of adding meaning ('access', *shingila*) to natural force (the herbal mixture obtained at that stage). His recipe actually talked to the environment. Through prefixes and suffixes added to a stem, Bantu languages can compose virtually any concept. Remember how the synonym for witch, *ng'wiboneeji*, was built up from morphemes. In the same way the magical recipe 'composes' its purpose. Each ingredient conveys a part of the message: naked at night, elephant, domestic water, roasted maize, potsherd and cross. The totality of medicinal morphemes, structured around the stem 'black roasted seeds' would more or less sound as follows: 'Through this magic secretly administered, any intruder of fields that belong to my house will incur the spell of my ancestors who joined forces at the threshold of my house'.

Language itself is a coupling of sounds (or some other sensory data) with meaning. The human organism has learned to experience the latter when perceiving the former. Magic is a special case where sensory data synaesthetically reinforces meaning so that the user's body, mind, and group undergoes a beneficial effect with its application. To savour the radiant potential of magical epistemology a brief theoretical excursion may be in order.

In her study of magic in contemporary Russia, Galina Lindquist (2004) courageously endeavoured to supplement her analysis of healing with a discussion that engages on equal terms with the epistemology of healing. As cultural outsiders we need not accept the literal claims of the healer, but after finding common ground we may come to an intercultural version of those claims and learn something new that enriches our epistemology. A first step in this exercise in cultural comparison was taken by Malinowski (1922) and later by Lévi-Strauss (1962). As Lindquist (2004: 170) notes, anthropologists have emphasized the importance of magical language; how expressions are instrumental. In the Peircean terms Lindquist adopts, 'ritual speech is more pragmatic than descriptive or referential, and, thus, it acts, primarily, iconically and indexically' (ibid.) She argues, furthermore, that the pragmatic is in the magic's affinity (Peircean 'community') with existing clusters of power. As we appreciated in divination, magic stages the unspeakable, even quite ugly emotions. Its invocation of these states attests to its mastery over the world. Through the participants' subjectivity, magic may be thought to subsequently influence those clusters (something which, as Lindquist reminds us, Tambiah and Csordas, among others, have pointed out). The next step in our rapprochement with the healer's epistemology goes a bit further for it asks to what extent we may assume the subjectivity of the non-participant to be affected, such as the countered witch or the attacked patient unaware of the magic administered. Lindquist (2004: 171) sums up the epistemology of a Russian healer: strings of uttered words would cause vibrations in the air at frequencies that interact with brain and body; these 'spells … accompanied by the requisite ritual actions, change the energy-information structures of the world and alter its physical and situational patterns in desired directions'. Willerslev (2007) and Holbraad (2007) are two authors among a growing number exploring how far ethnographers can (and perhaps should) go along with another culture's epistemology, given that at some point it will conflict with the beliefs of the ethnographer. This book has not defended the beliefs of Sukuma healers, but it has sympathized with their epistemology. The epistemology was not situated in determinate beliefs but in the experiential frames accompanying them. From that point I want to go deeper into the medical (hence as much material as semantic) implications of frames and their shifts.

David Parkin's recent remark about magic, in the context of holism, seems particularly fruitful for our discussion: medicinal herbs are curative but in some societies have to 'be persuaded to agree to become curative' (Parkin 2007: 11). That seems the point of the Sukuma healer's search for ingredients of 'access'. Agreement refers to the connectedness of the herbs to a larger whole. Our reflex is to find this magical or animist position 'superstitious', which may stem from our unspoken mechanistic concept of efficacy. A well-known illustration of our mechanistic inclination and of its detrimental bias is that antibiotics effectively treat isolated organisms but may harm self-healing capacities on a larger scale.

If, on the one hand, technology serves as an extension of our sensory apparatus, helping the body with those extensions to perceive more of the environment, reaching further, digging deeper for anything meaningful or useful to the body; and if, on the other hand, art starts from an intuition about the world and makes this imperceptible budding reality, a meaning out there, enter the body by affecting the observer's senses appropriately, then magic has something of both technology and art. A magical recipe seeks to expand the influence of the body on the world (including the spirit world) and vice versa: expand the influence of that world on the body. Magic affects the environment as much as it attests to a profound comprehension of the environment. Since world and environment are used here as holistic concepts – comprising nature, society and their residual unknown (as the reference to spirits indicates) – we accordingly understand the comprehension of world and environment as a holistic process; namely less as an unravelling of a passive object by a scientist or alchemist, and more as a coming to terms with, or (in Parkin's terms) finding 'agreement' with the world, recognizing the latter's active role in our understanding. Thus I understand Lindquist's point that the healer enters into (Peircean) community with the structure of the world.

Why do healers expect the body to get better by becoming one with the world? Why should a semantic structure make any difference for the patient's body? It is time we resume our discussion on the holistic approach. We have seen that healers do not think of meanings as mere signifiers in a symbolic order segregated from the real. Meanings are indissoluble from matter, hence can be good or bad for the body. Sukuma healers adopt more sophisticated (and no less comprehensive) structures than the binary good/bad: reciprocal, intrusive, expulsive and synchronous, to list the four this book discerned. A quaternary system suits diviners better than a judgemental binarism when having to switch perspectives between opponents in a feud, or having to deal with both white and black magic, and having to negotiate with possible witches so as to develop effective antidotes. The common opposition between white and black magic (with red in-between) eclipses the four dimensions of magic. As for the first dimension, in the way the user of magic operates, reciprocity predominates; the healer ventures into the forest to collect roots but also depends on dreams sent by the ancestral guide to find 'access'. Secondly, the lethal type of access is what witches obtain. The expulsive dimension of magic we find in ritual healing. The fourth dimension is the synchrony, or 'agreeing' mentioned earlier, which magic relies on. Spirits too exhibit these four dimensions: a reciprocal guide (for which many names are used: *isamva*, 'ancestral spirit', *ntale*, 'great one', *ndugu*, 'kin', *nkulugenji*, 'director', from the Swahili *mkurugenzi*), a provoked one (*ndagu*, 'curse', *njimu*, 'angry spirit', *nzoka*, 'snake', but also *isamva* in its etymology, cf. Chapter 5), an investigative eye (*liso*, also *nhebe*, 'canoe-seat', cf. Chapter 6) and a calling (*mahugi*, also *lusuutila*, 'stalker', *liyoka*, 'great snake').

Especially the fourth dimension of magic requires further elucidation. Therefore, let us for a moment return to Seele's patients suffering from *mayabu* after stepping on an invisible trap. Therapy over a period of one to two years causes the affliction to retreat downwardly. Part of the therapy, discussed in Chapter 2, is the medicine of the 'broom' (*ikumbo*). It induces acute diarrhoea to expel the mass of black magic, after which other remedies get the intestines settled again. The medicine's 'access' is the straw of an old broom. Obviously the straw links the medicine metonymically with the concept of a broom, which itself is a metaphor to invoke the desired outcome: cleaning. Metaphor has played a central role in the study of ritual and magic (Turner 1967; Fernandez 1982; Csordas 1994). Metaphors establish a connection between seemingly unrelated domains of life. As the 'meta' in metaphor suggests, the user (in a spell or a ritual) overcomes already existing limitations and achieves an unforeseen connection between semantic fields (Devisch 1993). An act of power takes place. The mistake, however, would be to locate the power in this creative moment, as if the metaphor is a mechanism generating healing. That has been the logic appreciated by cognitive scientists writing on metaphor (cf. Kövesces 2003). In my view the power of magic lies in the connection with the rest of the system. It responds to something already there, such as the threat called moral power. The broom means nothing by itself. It fits within a chain of associations comprising dirt in the house, cleaning, trouble in the family, ejection, feelings such as the comfort Albert got from sweeping the paths, and more, which derive their meaning from a certain frame of experience, differentiated from other frames healers are trained into. Now, to comprehend the fourth dimension, let us turn one last time to that rich source of inspiration that is a Bantu language.

From Richardson's (1966) linguistic study I inferred that the Sukuma word closest to metaphor is *shikolile*, which consists of the stem -*kola*, 'to resemble', and the suffix -*ile*, a morpheme commonly used to express 'in the presence of a third'. The object, a broom, does not in itself resemble cleaning. It does so in the eyes of a third, the subject – which sounds pretty wise, reflexive and (modernly) relativistic. Would subjective construction be the property of metaphors? When I discussed this with Paulo he did something important, which he often did: he disagreed. Metaphor, conceived in this way, would not be the point of magic or ritual. Moreover, he proposed another term, which he had heard among the healers he grew up with and considered more apt than *shikolile* to understand magical ingredients: *shikolanijo*. The word is difficult to translate. As noted before, Bantu languages allow for inventive construction. The word consists of the same stem as *shikolile*: -*kola*, 'to resemble', but it has a different suffix: -*anijo*, which is used to signify 'simultaneously'. Magic and intention resemble one another simultaneously, or in synchrony, and therefore magic works.

What could it mean that instead of 'resembling' a purpose (such as cleaning) and this (quite relativistically) 'in the eyes of the subject' (*shikolile*), the magical ingredient resembles it simultaneously (*shikolanijo*)? Might we be introduced here to a post-relativistic position? From the many discussions I had with Paulo afterwards, a few hypotheses can be drawn. First of all, magic does two things at once: resemble a thing (cleaning) and make the thing happen (rid the stomach of poison). Secondly, Paulo emphasized that magic does not always work. The right kind has to be applied at the right time, which is a matter of intuition, something healers specialize in (remember the dream needed to enter the forest, the required mark on the spleen before divination and initiation, or the vision entering before the diviner can drum to convoke the patient). Medicinal herbs have to 'agree' to become curative, as Parkin puts it. Tambiah's (1973) persuasive analogies, established by the ingredients as illustrated by forms of *shingila*, do not suffice. Paulo seemed to be objecting to the spatial slant of the metaphor concept, which places the subject beyond any specified place (meta) and in the position of creator (compare 'in the presence of a third' in *shikolile*) and 'referring to', hence transcending the world. It obscures the temporal dimension, that of the states (or places, topoi) the system can shift between over time. Metonymy and metaphor turn magical only when they reflect the actual state the world is in; when ingredient (object) and intention (subject) are synchronous with the whole, so that the systemic can do its work. Thanks to initiation one may improve one's transmodal capacity to differentiate states of the system and detect the real state. Divination has this element of training, to obtain results in return for invested effort. But a fundamental uncertainty remains, which we called sacrifice. The healer depends on the dream to dig up the roots. The diviner waits for the right moment to sound the drum. In pregnant silence all those present commence the oracle with one question on their mind: Will the ancestor's eye show itself? Only the positivist assumes to be divining nothing but a dead chicken, as Paulo prosaically put it.

In Sukuma culture, magic and ritual are thought to work if their meanings are somehow synchronous with the state of the world. Postmodern anthropologists should be careful not to use the concept of culture in a culturalist way, purifying meaning from natural impact, typically emphasizing how 'cultural' (as in contingently constructed) all meanings are, hence unwittingly downplaying local knowledge and actually using the concept of 'culture' against the local culture of magic. In my view the culture concept can also support the healer's claim of efficacy, for meanings are indissoluble from a particular situation, inhering in the matter used for the patient's recovery. The same meaning can be in the objects, the broom, the body, the neurons, if you will. Therefore, to signal the exploration I began in Chapter 2, I propose a term – a last one – to elicit this efficacy of magic: synaesthetics. Magic exploits the systemic in defiance of modal segregations such as mind and body (see also Stroeken 2008b). Magic is synaesthetic, as the desired bodily and social outcome gets coupled with the inserted meaningful ingredient, much like clinical synaesthesia wherein a mood or the sight of a colour follows the hearing of a certain sound.

That is why healing in Bantu cultures amounts to initiation, and throughout this book I have insisted on this aspect of meaning. Patients have to be initiated into a medicine; they have to be imbued with the meanings inhering in the matter, such as the roots and bark they will have regularly dug up and ground, and that they will have administered to other patients, and perhaps they will have dreamt. A culture disposes to certain couplings. Ritual initiation as well as long-term training at a healer's compound reinforces the coupling of magic with a certain state. Nobody can really know another person's experience. But I hope to have shown that the rituals 'know' the *structures* of those experiences. Those structures point to states and their shifts.

The intercultural exercise of this book has to a considerable extent been the product of my personal *Chwezi* experience. *Chwezi* novices were not taught religious beliefs; they came to experience states. The question remains how those states we were initiated into could have a sensory ground and at the same time so well translate into the various forms of social exchange that keep society together. How can the visceral be moral? It will take a more collective effort than mine here to further explore this post-Kantian matter.

# Notes

1. *Natula buganga wane wa ndagu. Unene Ichaniki nang'witanaga umuna Ndagu, uwitanilwa aha kaya yane na mili gwane. Ihaha nakufunya aha mili nakuleke aha nzilamaka nulu unshokele uyo wa kutuma unogi wako. Unene nakufunyaga uje mu nyanza ukaliwe mang'wiina na Masanza gwina. Fumaga ukachiile mu nyanza, uje, ng'wa Luhinda.*

249

# References

Abrahams, R.G. 1967. *The Peoples of Greater Unyamwezi*. London: International African Institute.

———. 1987. 'Sungusungu: Village Vigilante Groups in Tanzania', *African Affairs* 343: 179–96.

———. (ed.) 1994. *Witchcraft in Contemporary Tanzania*. Cambridge: African Studies Centre.

Alexander, J. 2003. *The Meanings of Social Life: A Cultural Sociology*. Oxford: Oxford University Press.

Appadurai, A. 1986. 'Commodities and the Politics of Value', in A. Appadurai (ed.) *The Social Life of Things*. Cambridge: Cambridge University Press.

———. 1996. *Modernity At Large*. Minneapolis: University of Minnesota Press.

Appiah, K.A. 1993. *In My Father's House: Africa in the Philosophy of Culture*. New York: Oxford University Press.

Ashforth, A. 2000. *Madumo: A Man Bewitched*. Chicago: Chicago University Press.

———. 2001. 'On Living in a World with Witches', in H. Moore and T. Sanders (eds), *Magical Interpretations, Material Realities*. New York: Routledge.

Augé, M. 1975. 'Logique lignagère et logique de Bregbo', in C. Piault (ed.) *Prophétisme et thérapeutique: Albert Atcho et la communauté de Bregbo*. Paris: Editions Hermann.

Auslander, M. 1993. '"Open the Wombs!": The Symbolic Politics of Modern Ngoni Witchfinding', in J. and J. Comaroff (ed.) *Modernity and its Malcontents*. Chicago: University of Chicago Press.

Badiou, A. 2005. *Being and Event*. New York: Continuum.

Bataille, G. 1991. *The Accursed Share, Volume 1: Consumption*. Cambridge: MIT Press.

Bateson, G. 1990[1972]. *Steps to an Ecology of Mind*. New York: Ballantine.

Batibo, H. 1985. *Le Kesukuma: Phonologie, Morphologie*. Paris: Editions de la Recherche sur les Civilisations.

Baudrillard, J. 1994. *Simulacra and Simulation*. Ann Arbor: Michigan University Press.

Bayart, J.-F. 1993. *The State in Africa: The Politics of the Belly*. London: Longman.

Beck, U., A. Giddens and S. Lash. 1994. *Reflexive Modernization: Politics, Tradition and Aesthetics in the Modern Social Order.* Cambridge: Polity Press.

Beidelman, T.O. 1986. *Moral Imagination in Kaguru Modes of Thought.* Bloomington: Indiana University Press.

Binsbergen, W. van. 1991. 'Becoming a Sangoma: Religious Anthropological Fieldwok in Francistown, Botswana', *Journal of Religion in Africa* 21(4): 308–44.

––––––. 2003. *Intercultural Encounters: African and Anthropological Lessons Towards a Philosophy of Interculturality.* Berlin: LIT.

Birchwood, M. and P. Trower. 2006. 'The Future of Cognitive-behavioural Therapy for Psychosis: Not a Quasi-neuroleptic', *British Journal of Psychiatry* 188: 107–8.

Boddy, J. 1989. *Wombs and Alien Spirits: Women, Men and the Zar in Northern Sudan.* Madison: University of Winsconsin Press.

––––––. 1994. 'Spirit Possession Revisited: Beyond Instrumentality', *Annual Review of Anthropology* 23: 407–434.

Bond, G. and D. Ciekawy. 2001. 'Contested Domains in the Dialogues of "Witchcraft"', in C. Bond and D. Ciekawy (eds), *Witchcraft Dialogues: Anthropological and Philosophical Exchanges.* Athens: Ohio University Press.

Bösch, F. 1930. *Les Banyamwezi, Peuple de l'Afrique Orientale.* Münster: Bibliotheca Africana.

Bourdieu, P. 1979. *La Distinction: Critique Sociale du Jugement.* Paris: Minuit.

––––––. 1980. *Le Sens Pratique.* Paris: Minuit.

Brandström, P. 1990. 'Seeds and Soil: The Quest for Life and the Domestication of Fertility in Sukuma Thought and Reality', in A. Jacobson-Widding and W. van Beek (eds), *The Creative Communion: African Folk Models of Fertility and the Regeneration of Life.* Uppsala: Alqvist and Wiksell.

––––––. 1991. 'Boundless Universe: The Culture of Expansion Among the Sukuma-Nyamwezi People'. Ph.D. dissertation. Uppsala: Uppsala University.

Cheal, D. 1988. *The Gift Economy.* London: Routledge.

Clifford, J. 1988. *The Predicament of Culture: Twentieth Century Ethnography, Literature, and Art.* Cambridge, MA: Harvard University Press.

Comaroff, J. 1985. *Body of Power, Spirit of Resistance: The Culture and History of a South African People.* Chicago: Chicago University Press.

Comaroff, J. and J.L. Comaroff. 1993. 'Introduction', in J. and J.L. Comaroff (eds), *Modernity and its Malcontents.* Chicago: University of Chicago Press.

––––––. 2000. 'Millennial Capitalism: First Thoughts on a Second Coming', *Public Culture* 12: 291–343.

Cory, H. 1949. 'The Ingredients of Magic Medicines', *Africa* 19(1): 13–32.

———. 1953. *Sukuma Law and Custom*. London: Oxford University Press.

———. 1955. 'The Buswezi', *American Anthropologist* 57(5): 923–52.

Crapanzano, V. 1977. 'Introduction', in V. Crapanzano and V. Garrison (eds), *Case Studies in Spirit Possession*. New York: John Wiley.

Csordas, T. 1994. 'Introduction', in T. Csordas (ed.) *Embodiment and Experience: The Existential Ground of Culture and Self*. Cambridge: Cambridge University Press.

———. 1996. 'Imaginal Performance and Memory in Ritual Healing', in C. Laderman and M. Roseman (eds), *The Performance of Healing*. New York: Routledge.

DeLanda, M. 2006. *A New Philosophy of Society: Assemblage Theory and Social Complexity*. New York: Continuum.

Derrida, J. 1992. *Given Time, Volume I: Counterfeit Money*. Chicago: University of Chicago Press.

Descombes, V. 2001. *The Mind's Provisions: A Critique of Cognitivism*. Princeton, NJ: Princeton University Press.

Devisch, R. 1993. *Weaving the Threads of Life: The Khita Gyn-Eco-Logical Healing Cult among the Yaka*. Chicago: Chicago University Press.

Douglas, M. 1970. 'Introduction', in M. Douglas (ed.) *Witchcraft Confessions and Accusations*. London: Tavistock.

———. 1994. *Risk and Blame: Essays in Cultural Theory*. London: Routledge.

Doyle, S. 2007. 'The Cwezi-Kubandwa Debate: Gender, Hegemony and Pre-colonial Religion in Bunyoro, Western Uganda', *Africa* 77(4): 559–81.

Dumont, Louis. 1986. *Essays on Individualism: Modern Ideology in Anthropological Perspective*. Chicago: University of Chicago Press.

EIU. 1998. *Tanzania: Country Profile 1998–99*. New York: Economist Intelligence Unit.

Englund, Harri. 1996. 'Witchcraft, Modernity and the Person: The Morality of Accumulation in Central Malawi', *Critique of Anthropology* 16: 257–79.

———. 2002. 'Ethnography after Globalism: Migration and Emplacement in Malawi', *American Ethnologist* 29: 261–86

Evans-Pritchard, E.E. 1976[1937]. *Witchcraft, Oracle and Magic among the Azande*. Oxford: Oxford University Press.

Evens, T.M.S., and D. Handelman. 2006. *The Manchester School: Practice and Ethnographic Praxis in Anthropology*. Oxford: Berghahn Books.

Fabian, J. 1983. *Time and the Other: How Anthropology Makes its Objects*. New York: Columbia University Press.

Farelius, B. 2008. *Origins of Kingship: Traditions and Symbolism in the Great Lakes Region of Africa*. Uppsala: Acta Universitatis Upsaliensis.

Favret-Saada, J. 1980. *Deadly Words: Witchcraft in the Bocage*. New York: Cambridge University Press.

Feenberg, A. 1998. *Questioning Technology*. New York: Routledge.

Fernandez, J. 1982. *Bwiti: An Ethnography of the Religious Imagination in Africa*. Princeton, NJ: Princeton University Press.

Fisiy, C. and P. Geschiere. 2001. 'Witchcraft, Development and Paranoia in Cameroon', in H. Moore and T. Sanders, *Magical Interpretations, Material Realities*. New York: Routledge.

Foucault, M. 1975. *The Birth of the Clinic: An Archaeology of Medical Perception*. New York: Vintage.

———. 2001. *The Order of Things: An Archaeology of the Human Sciences*. London: Routledge.

Gadamer, H.G. 2004. *Truth and Method*. London: Continuum.

Gaonkar, D. 1999. 'On Alternative Modernities', *Public Culture* 11: 1–18.

Geertz, C. 1973. *The Interpretation of Cultures*. London: Fontana.

Gellner, E. 1992. *Reason and Culture*. Oxford: Blackwell.

Geschiere, P. 1997. *The Modernity of Witchcraft: Politics and the Occult in Postcolonial Africa*. Charlottesville: University of Virginia Press.

Girard, R. 1993. *Things Hidden Since the Foundation of the World*. Stanford, CA: Stanford University Press.

Gluckman, M. 1970[1956]. *Custom and Conflict in Africa*. Oxford: Blackwell.

Godbout, J. 1992. *L'esprit du don*. Paris: La Découverte.

Goffman, E. 1974. *Frame Analysis: An Essay on the Organisation of Experience*. Harmondsworth: Penguin.

Green, M. 2005. 'Discourses on Inequality', *Anthropological Theory* 5: 247–66.

Green, M. and S. Mesaki. 2005. 'The Birth of the "Salon": Poverty, 'Modernization', and Dealing with Witchcraft in Southern Tanzania', *American Ethnologist* 32: 371–88.

Gregory, C. 1982. *Gifts and Commodities*. London: Academic Press.

Griaule, M. 1975. *Conversations with Ogotemmeli: An Introduction to Dogon Religious Ideas*. Oxford: Oxford University Press.

Griaule, M. and G. Dieterlen. 1986. *The Pale Fox*. Chino Valley: Continuum foundation.

Grosz, E. 1990. *Jacques Lacan: A Feminist Introduction*. London: Routledge.

Gunderson, F.D. 2001. 'From "Dancing with Porcupines" to "Twirling a Hoe": Musical Labor Transformed in Sukumaland, Tanzania', *Africa Today* 48(4): 3–25.

Habermas, J. 1985. *The Theory of Communicative Action, Volume 1: Reason and the Rationalization of Society*. New York: Beacon.

Handelman, D. 1998. *Models and Mirrors: Towards an Anthropology of Public Events*. New York: Berghahn Books.

Hendriks, J. 1988. 'Shingwengwe', in M. Tertrais (ed.), *Imani za Jadi za Kisukuma*. Mwanza: Bujora Sukuma Research Committee.

Herzfeld, M. 2001. *Anthropology: Theoretical Practice in Culture and Society.* London: Blackwell.

Heusch, Luc de. 1966. *Le Rwanda et la Civilisation Interlacustre.* Bruxelles: Université Libre de Bruxelles.

———. 1985. *Sacrifice in Africa: A Structuralist Approach.* Manchester: Manchester University Press.

———. 1995. 'Rwanda: Responsibilities for a Genocide', *Anthropology Today* 11: 3–7.

Holbraad, Martin. 2007. 'The Power of Powder: Multiplicity and Motion in the Divinatory Cosmology of Cuban Ifá (or Mana, again)', in A. Henare, M. Holbraad and S. Wastell (eds), *Thinking Through Things: Theorising Artefacts Ethnographically.* London: Routledge.

Holy, L. 1987. 'Description, Generalisation and Comparison: Two Paradigms', in L. Holy (ed.) *Comparative Anthropology.* Oxford: Blackwell.

Hountondji, P. 1983. *African Philosophy: Myth and Reality.* Bloomington: Indiana University Press.

Horton, R. 1967. 'African Traditional Thought and Western Science', *Africa* 37: 50–71, 155–87.

Howell, S. 1996. 'Introduction', in S. Howell (ed.), *For the Sake of Our Future: Sacrificing in Eastern Indonesia.* Leiden: CNWS.

Howes, D. 2003. *Sensual Relations: Engaging the Senses in Culture and Social Theory.* Ann Arbor: University of Michigan Press.

Hubert, H. and M. Mauss. 1899. 'Essai sur la Nature et la Fonction du Sacrifice', *Année Sociologique* 2: 29–138.

Hyden, G. 1980. *Beyond Ujamaa in Tanzania: Underdevelopment and an Uncaptured Peasantry.* London: Heinemann.

Ingold, T. 2000. *The Perception of the Environment.* New York: Routledge.

Israel, J. 2001. *The Radical Enlightenment: Philosophy and the Making of Modernity, 1650–1750.* Oxford: Oxford University Press.

Jackson, M. 1989. *Paths Toward a Clearing: Radical Empiricism and Ethnographic Enquiry.* Bloomington: Indiana University Press.

Jackson, M. and I. Karp (eds.). 1990. *Personhood and Agency: The Experience of Self and Other in African Cultures.* Stockholm: Almqvist and Wiksell.

Jameson, F. 1991. *Postmodernism: Or, The Cultural Logic of Late Capitalism.* London: Verso.

Janzen, J.M. 1992. *Ngoma: Discourses of Healing in Central and Southern Africa.* Berkeley: University of California Press.

Kapferer, B. 1997. *The Feast of the Sorcerer: Practices of Consciousness and Power.* Chicago: University of Chicago Press.

———. 2003. 'Outside All Reason', in B. Kapferer (ed.) *Beyond Rationalism: Rethinking Magic, Witchcraft and Sorcery.* Oxford: Berghahn Books.

Kaptchuk, T.J. 2002. 'The Placebo Effect in Alternative Medicine: Can the Performance of a Healing Ritual Have Clinical Significance?' *Annals of Internal Medicine* 136(11): 817–25.

Karp, I. 1980. 'Beer Drinking and Social Experience in an African Society', in I. Karp and C. Bird (eds.) *Explorations in African Systems of Thought.* Bloomington: Indiana University Press.

Kelly, R. 1976. 'Witchcraft and Sexual Relations: An Exploration of the Social and Semantic Implications of the Structure of Belief', in P. Brown and G. Buchbinder (eds.) *Man and Woman in the New Guinea Highlands.* Washington, DC: American Anthropological Association.

Kirmayer, L.J. and N. Sartorius. 2007. 'Cultural Models and Somatic Syndromes', *Psychosomatic Medicine* 69: 832–40.

Knauft, B. 2007. 'Moral Exchange and Exchanging Morals: Alternative Paths of Cultural Change in Papua New Guinea', in J. Barker (ed.) *The Anthropology of Morality in Melanesia and Beyond.* Burlington, VT: Ashgate.

Kövecses, Z. 2003. *Metaphor and Emotion: Language, Culture and Body in Human Feeling.* Cambridge: Cambridge University Press.

Lacan, J. 1973. *Le Séminaire, livre XI: les quatre concepts fondamentaux de la psychanalyse, 1964.* Paris: Seuil.

Lakoff, G. and M. Johnson. 1980. *Metaphors We Live By.* Chicago: Chicago University Press.

Lambek, M. 1993. *Knowledge and Practice in Mayotte: Local Discourses of Islam, Sorcery, and Spirit Possession.* Toronto: University of Toronto Press.

Latour, B. 1993. *We Have Never Been Modern.* London: Harvester.

Lattas, A. 1998. *Cultures of Secrecy: Reinventing Race in Bush Kaliai Cargo Cults.* Madison: University of Wisconsin Press.

Lespinay, C. de. 2001. 'The Churches and the Genocide in the East African Great Lakes Region', in O. Bartov and P. Mack (eds), *In God's Name: Genocide and Religion in the Twentieth Century.* Oxford: Berghahn Books.

Lévi-Strauss, C. 1949. *Les Structures elémentaires de la parenté.* Paris: Presses Universtaires de France.

_____. 1962. *La Pensée sauvage.* Paris: Plon.

_____. 1972. *Structural Anthropology I.* London: Penguin Books.

Lienhardt, G. 1970. *Divinity and Experience: The Religion of the Dinka.* Oxford: Clarendon Press.

Lindquist, G. 2004. *Conjuring Hope: Magic and Healing in Contemporary Russia.* Oxford: Berghahn Books.

Longman, T. 2001. 'Christian Churches and Genocide in Rwanda', in O. Bartov and P. Mack (eds), *In God's Name: Genocide and Religion in the Twentieth Century.* Oxford: Berghahn Books.

Lopez, S.R. and P.J. Guarnaccia. 2000. 'Cultural Psychopathology: Uncovering the Social World of Mental Illness', *Annual Review of Psychology* 51: 571–98.

Luhmann, N. 1995. *Social Systems*. Stanford, CA: Stanford University Press.

Luhrman, T. 1989. *Persuasions of the Witch's Craft*. Cambridge, MA: Harvard University Press.

Macfarlane, A. 1999. *Witchcraft in Tudor and Stuart England*. London: Routledge.

Mcintosh, J. 2004. 'Reluctant Muslims: Embodied Hegemony and Moral Resistance in a Giriama Spirit Possession Complex', *Journal of the Royal Anthropological Institute* 10: 91–112.

Malinowski, B. 1922. *Argonauts of the Western Pacific*. London: Routledge and Kegan Paul.

Malkki, L. 1995. *Purity and Exile: Violence, Memory, and National Cosmology Among Hutu Refugees in Tanzania*. Chicago: University of Chicago Press.

Marcus, G. and M. Fischer. 1986. *Anthropology as Cultural Critique: An Experimental Moment in the Human Sciences*. Chicago: University of Chicago Press.

Marwick, M. 1952. 'The Social Context of Cewa Witch Beliefs', *Africa* 22: 120–35.

———. 1970. 'Introduction', in M. Marwick (ed.) *Witchcraft and Sorcery*. London: Penguin.

Mauss, M. 1974[1925]. *The Gift*. London: Routledge.

Mbembe, A. 2001. *On the Postcolony*. Berkeley: University of California Press.

Mesaki, S. 1994. 'Witch-killing in Sukumaland', in R. Abrahams (ed.) *Witchcraft in Contemporary Tanzania*. Cambridge: African Studies Centre.

Meyer, B. and P. Pels. 2003. *Magic and Modernity: Interfaces of Revelation and Concealment*. Stanford, CA: Stanford University Press.

Middleton, J. 1963. 'Witchcraft and Sorcery in Lugbara', in J. Middleton and E. Winter (eds), *Witchcraft and Sorcery in East Africa*. London: Routledge and Kegan Paul.

Miguel, E. 2005. 'Poverty and Witch Killing in Tanzania', *Review of Economic Studies* 72: 1153–72.

Milbank, J. 1995. 'Stories of Sacrifice: From Wellhausen to Girard', *Theory, Culture and Society* 12(4): 15–46.

Millroth, B. 1965. *Lyuba, Traditional Religion of the Sukuma*. Uppsala: Almqvist and Wiksell.

Mitchell, J.C. 1956. *The Yao Village: A Study in the Social Structure of a Nyasaland Tribe*. Manchester: Manchester University Press.

Mitchell, P. 2005. *African Connections: An Archaeological Perspective on Africa and the Wider World*. New York: Rowman Altamira.

Moerman, D. 2002. *Meaning, Medicine, and 'the Placebo Effect'*. Cambridge: Cambridge University Press.

Moore, H. and T. Sanders. 2001. 'Magical Interpretations and Material Realities,' in H. Moore and T. Sanders (eds), *Magical Interpretations, Material Realities*. New York: Routledge.

Mudimbe, V. 1988. *The Invention of Africa: Gnosis, Philosophy, and the Order of Knowledge*. Bloomington: Indian University Press.

Needham, R. 1975. 'Polythetic Classification: Convergence and Consequences', *Man* 10(3): 349–69.

Neu, J. 1970. 'Lévi-Strauss on Shamanism', *Man* 10: 285–92.

Niehaus, I. 2001a. *Witchcraft, Power and Politics: Exploring the Occult in the South African Lowveld*. London: Pluto.

———. 2001b. 'Witchcraft in the New South Africa: From Colonial Superstition to Post-colonial Reality?' in H. Moore and T. Sanders (eds), *Magical Interpretations, Material Realities*. New York: Routledge.

Nyamnjoh, F. 2001. 'Delusions of Development and the Enrichment of Witchcraft Discourses in Cameroon', in H. Moore and T. Sanders (eds), *Magical Interpretations, Material Realities*. New York: Routledge.

Nyanchama-Okemwa, S. 2002. 'Rhetoric of Remembrance: Privileged Authority and the Contested Gradations of Seniority,' in S. Makoni and K. Stroeken (eds), *Ageing in Africa*. Aldershot: Ashgate.

Ortigues, C. and E. Ortigues. 1966. *Œdipe Africain*. Paris: Plon.

Ortner, S. 2006. *Anthropology and Social Theory: Culture, Power, and the Acting Subject*. Durham, NC: Duke University Press.

Overing, J. 1987. 'Translation as a Creative Process: The Power of the Name', in L. Holy (ed.) *Comparative Anthropology*. Oxford: Blackwell.

Parker, J. 2004. 'Witchcraft, Anti-witchcraft and Trans-regional Ritual Innovation In Early Colonial Ghana: Sakrabundi and Aberewa, 1889–1910', *Journal of African History* 45(3): 393–420.

Parkin, D. 1985. 'Entitling Evil: Muslims and Non-Muslims in Coastal Kenya', in D. Parkin (ed.) *The Anthropology of Evil*. Oxford: Blackwell.

——— 2007. 'Introduction: Emergence and Convergence', in D. Parkin and S. Ulijascek (eds), *Holistic Anthropology: Emergence and Convergence*. Oxford: Berghahn Books.

Parry, J. 1986. 'The Gift, the Indian Gift and the "Indian Gift"', *Man* 21: 453–73.

Parry, J. and M. Bloch. 1989. 'Introduction: Money and the Morality of Exchange', in J. Parry and M. Bloch (eds), *Money and the Morality of Exchange*. Cambridge: Cambridge University Press.

Peek, P. 1991. 'Introduction', in P. Peek (ed.) *African Divination Systems: Ways of Knowing*. Bloomington: Indiana University Press.

Peer, J. et al. 2007. 'Identifying Mechanisms of Treatment Effects and Recovery in Rehabilitation of Schizophrenia: Longitudinal Analytic Methods', *Clinical Psychology Review* 27(6): 696–714.

Pels, P. and L. Nencel. 1991. 'Critique and the Deconstruction of Anthropological Authority', in L. Nencel and P. Pels (eds), *Constructing Knowledge: Authority and Critique in Social Science*. London: Sage.

Pred, A. and M.J. Watts. 1992. *Reworking Modernity: Capitalisms and Symbolic Discontent*. New Brunswick, NJ: Rutgers University Press.

Ranger, T.O. 1975. *Dance and Society in Eastern Africa, 1890–1970: The Beni Ngoma*. Berkeley: University of California Press.

———. 2007. 'Scotland Yard in the Bush: Medicine Murders, Child Witches and the Construction of the Occult: A Literature Review', *Africa* 77: 272–83.

Richardson, I. 1966. 'A Vocabulary of Sukuma', in W.M. Mann (ed.) *African Language Studies, VII: Collected Papers in Oriental and African Studies*. London: Luzac and Co.

Ricoeur, P. 1991. *From Text to Action: Essays in Hermeneutics II*. London: Athlone.

Rivera, D. et al. 2003. 'Review of Food and Medicinal Uses of Capparis L. Subgenus Capparis (Capparidaceae)', *Economic Botany* 57(4): 515–34.

Rorty, R. 1989. *Contingency, Irony, and Solidarity*. Cambridge: Cambridge University Press.

Rutherford, B. 1999. 'To Find an African Witch: Anthropology, Modernity, and Witch-finding in North-west Zimbabwe', *Critique of Anthropology* 19(1): 89–109.

Sahlins, M. 1976. *Culture and Practical Reason*. Chicago: Chicago University Press.

———. 1999. 'Two or Three Things That I Know about Culture', *Journal of the Royal Anthropological Institute* 5: 399–421.

Sanders, T. 2001. 'Save Our Skins: Structural Adjustment, Morality and the Occult in Tanzania', in H. Moore and T. Sanders (eds), *Magical Interpretations, Material Realities*. New York: Routledge.

Sargent, C. 1989. *Maternity, Medicine, and Power: Reproductive Decisions in Urban Benin*. Berkeley: University of California Press.

Schwartz, J. 2002. *The Mind and The Brain: Neuroplasticity and the Power of Mental Force*. New York: HarperCollins.

Searle, J. 2006. 'Social Ontology: Some Basic Principles', *Anthropological Theory* 6: 12–29.

Shipton, P. 1989. *Bitter Money: Cultural Economy and Some African Meanings of Forbidden Commodities*. Washington, DC: American Ethnological Society.

Schoeneman, T.J. 1975. 'The Witch Hunt as a Culture Change Phenomenon', *Ethos* 3: 529–54.

Siegel, J. 2006. *Naming The Witch*. Stanford, CA: Stanford University Press.

Solms, M. 2004. 'Freud Returns', *Scientific American* 290 (5): 82–88.

Sörensen, Jesper. 2006. *A Cognitive Theory of Magic*. New York: Altamira.

Spaulding, W.D. 1997. 'Cognitive Models in a Fuller Understanding of Schizophrenia', *Psychiatry* 60(4): 341–46.

Spencer-Brown, G. 1969. *Laws of Form*. London: Allen and Unwin.

Spivak, G. 1988. *In Other Worlds: Essays in Cultural Politics*. London: Routledge.

Sternberg, M. 2000. *The Balance Within: The Science Connecting Health and Emotions*. New York: W.H. Freeman.

Stewart, P. and A. Strathern. 2004. *Witchcraft, Sorcery, Rumours and Gossip*. Cambridge: Cambridge University Press.

Stoller, P. 1989. *The Taste of Ethnographic Things: The Senses In Anthropology*. Philadelphia: University of Pennsylvania Press.

Strathern, A. and M. Lambek. 1998. 'Embodying Sociality: Africanist–Melanesianist Comparisons', in M. Lambek and A. Strathern, *Bodies and Persons*. Cambridge: Cambridge University Press.

Strauss, J.S. 1989. 'Mediating Processes in Schizophrenia: Towards a New Dynamic Psychiatry', *British Journal of Psychiatry* 169 (5): 22–28.

Stroeken, K. 2001. 'Defying the Gaze: Exodelics for the Bewitched in Sukumaland and Beyond', *Dialectical Anthropology* 26: 281–305.

———. 2002. 'From Shrub to Log: The Ancestral Dimension of Elderhood among Sukuma in Tanzania', in S. Makoni and K. Stroeken (eds), *Ageing in Africa: Sociolinguistic and Anthropological Approaches*. Aldershot: Ashgate.

———. 2004. 'In Search of the Real: The Healing Contingency of Sukuma Divination', in M. Winkelman and P. Peek (eds), *Divination and Healing: Potent Vision*. Tucson: University of Arizona Press.

———. 2005. 'Immunising Strategies: Hip Hop and Critique in Tanzania', *Africa* 75 (4): 488–509.

———. 2006. '"Stalking the Stalker": A Chwezi Initiation into Spirit Possession and Experiential Structure', *Journal of the Royal Anthropological Institute* 12(4): 785–802.

———. 2008a. 'Believed Belief: Science/Religion versus Sukuma Magic', *Social Analysis* 52(1): 144–65.

———. 2008b. 'Sensory Shifts and "Synaesthetics" in Sukuma Healing', *Ethnos* 73(4): 466–84.

Sumathipala, A., et al. 2004. 'Culture-bound Syndromes: The Story of *Dhat* Syndrome', *British Journal of Psychiatry* 184: 200–209.

Tambiah, S. 1973. 'Form and Meaning of Magical Acts: A Point of View', in R. Horton and R. Finnegan (eds), *Modes of Thought*. London: Faber.

_____. 1990. *Magic, Science, Religion and the Scope of Rationality*. Cambridge: Cambridge University Press.

Tanner, R.E.S. 1967. *Transition in African Beliefs: A Study in Sukumaland, Tanzania*. New York: Maryknoll Publications.

_____. 1970. *The Witch Murders in Sukumaland: A Sociological Commentary*. Uppsala: Nordiska Afrikainstitutet.

Taussig, M. 1980. *The Devil and Commodity Fetishism in South America*. Chapel Hill: University of North Carolina Press.

Taylor, Charles. 2004. *Modern Social Imaginaries*. Durham: Duke University Press.

Taylor, Christopher. 1999. *Sacrifice as Terror: The Rwandan Genocide of 1994*. Oxford: Berg.

Tcherkézoff, S. 1983. *Le Roi nyamwezi, la droite et la gauche: révision comparative des classifications dualistes*. Cambridge: Cambridge University Press.

_____. 1985. 'The Expulsion of Illness or the Domestication of the Dead: A Case Study of the Nyamwezi of Tanzania', *History and Anthropology* 2(1): 59–92.

Tseng, W.-S. 2006. 'From Peculiar Psychiatric Disorders through Culture-bound Syndromes to Culture-related Specific Syndromes', *Transcultural Psychiatry* 43(4): 554–76.

Turner, E. 2004. 'Drumming, Divination, and Healing: The Community at Work', in M. Winkelman and P. Peek (eds), *Divination and Healing: Potent Vision*. Tuscon: University of Arizona Press.

Turner, V. 1967. *The Forest of Symbols*. Ithaca, NY: Cornell University Press.

_____. 1968. *Schism and Continuity in an African Society*. Manchester: Manchester University Press.

_____. 1975. *Revelation and Divination in Ndembu Ritual*. Ithaca, NY: Cornell University Press.

Vansina, J. 2004. *Antecedents to Modern Rwanda: The Nyiginya Kingdom*. London: James Currey.

Varkevisser, C. 1973. *Socialisation in a Changing Society: Sukuma Childhood in Rural and Urban Mwanza, Tanzania*. The Hague: CESO.

Viveiros de Castro, E. 2004. 'Exchanging Perspectives: The Transformation of Objects into Subjects in Amerindian Ontologies', *Common Knowledge* 10(3): 463–84.

Waters, T. 1997. 'Beyond Structural Adjustment: State and Market in a Rural Tanzanian Village', *African Studies Review* 2: 59–89.

Weber, Max. 2002[1905]. *The Protestant Ethic and the Spirit of Capitalism*. New York: Penguin.

Werbner, R. 1989. *Ritual Passage, Sacred Journey: The Process and Organisation of Religious Movement*. Washington: Smithsonian Institution Press.

West, H. 2007. *Ethnographic Sorcery*. Chicago: University of Chicago Press.

Whyte, S.R. 1997. *Questioning Misfortune: The Pragmatics of Uncertainty in Eastern Uganda*. Cambridge: Cambridge University Press.

Wijsen, F.J.S. 1993. *There is Only One God: A Social-scientific and Theological Study of Popular Religion and Evangelization in Sukumaland, Northwest Tanzania*. Kampen: Kok.

Willerslev, R. 2007. *Soul Hunters: Hunting, Animism, and Personhood Among the Siberian Yukaghirs*. Berkeley: University of California Press.

Williams, R. 1975. *The Country and the City*. Oxford: Oxford University Press.

Willis, R.G. 1970. 'Instant Millennium: The Sociology of African Witch-cleansing Cults', in M. Douglas (ed.) *Witchcraft Confessions and Accusations*. London: Tavistock.

————. 1999. *Some Spirits Heal, Others Only Dance: A Journey into Human Selfhood in an African Village*. Oxford: Berg.

Wilson, M. 1951. 'Witch Beliefs and Social Structure', *American Journal of Sociology* 56: 307–13.

Wiredu, K. et al. (eds). 2004. *A Companion to African Philosophy*. Oxford: Blackwell.

Yamba, C.B. 1997. 'Cosmologies in Turmoil: Witchfinding and AIDS in Chiawa, Zambia', *Africa* 67(2): 200–223.

Zachar, P. 2000. 'Psychiatric Disorders Are Not Natural Kinds',?*Philosophy, Psychiatry and Psychology* 7(3): 167–82.

Zempléni, A. 1975. 'De la persécution à la culpabilité', in C. Piault (ed.) *Prophétisme et thérapeutique: Albert Atcho et la communauté de Bregbo*. Paris: Editions Hermann.

# Index